# WHEE for Wholistic Healing

# WORKBOOK

## Whole Health - Easily and Effectively

### AKA
### Wholistic Hybrid derived from EMDR and EFT

## Daniel J. Benor, MD, ABHM

Published by
Wholistic Healing Publications
P.O. Box 502
Medford, NJ 08055
www.WholisticHealingResearch.com
service@WholHealPubs.com

Printed in the United States of America

Revised 4/25/06

This workbook is printed on single sides of pages so that you will have plenty of room to write down your exercises on the facing blank pages as needed.

ISBN:
10 digit: 0-9754248-7-4
13 digit: 978-0-9754248-7-2

**Disclaimer:** *The techniques described in this e-book are intended as information for therapists, not for self-treatment. If you are having stress problems, you should seek the help of a therapist who can guide you in identifying and using the techniques that will best suit your problems.*

# Contents

## INTRODUCTION

*Our remedies oft in ourselves do lie.*
– William Shakespeare
*All's Well That Ends Well*

Self-healing can offer enormous benefits for physical and psychological problems. We can explore many avenues for dealing with our symptoms and issues through the many paths to self-healing presented in this manual.

Western society generally addresses the body as a physical thing to be treated mechanically and biochemically. Wholistic medicine views the body as an intimate part of our entire being, a participant in our emotional, mental, relational and spiritual life. Our inner self may speak to us through our body – for instance, when tensions are building up in our mind or relationships and we start to get headaches, backaches or stomach cramps. Listening to our bodymind when it speaks to us in such ways can help us de-stress.

Our body, emotions, mind, relationships (with other people and with your environment) and spirit all work together in a wholistic manner to create the state of health we are experiencing. Some of the self-healing methods described below are designed to address one or another of these levels; others invite engagement on all of them. A shift on any one level can facilitate wholistic shifts on all of the others. When we relax physically, we will have an easier time relaxing mentally and emotionally. When we meditate, we focus and discipline our mind; we also relax, learn to choose when and how much to engage our awareness with our emotions, and may open to spiritual awareness and healing. Being open to changing on all levels and using healing practices to help access our resources on each level can markedly facilitate our self-healing.

Our mind is an amazing biological computer that contains inner knowledge and stores memories of what is going on inside us. We know through our unconscious mind what is going on inside ourselves. This manual provides ways to get in touch with this inner wisdom, to explore and explain what is going on in our lives and to help us find the best ways to deal with our dis-ease and disease.

We are made of atoms and chemicals, but we also have biological energies that guide our inner processes. Einstein pointed this out, early in the last century. Modern physics has confirmed that this is correct. Matter and

4

NOTES

energies are actually two sides of the same thing. Conventional medicine has been very slow to absorb that our bodies can be understood and treated as energy. Wholistic healing also helps through energy medicine, the art and science of biological energies (bioenergies).

For more on the inter-relationships of spirit, relationships (with people and the environment, mind, emotions and body see
http://wholistichealingresearch.com/srmeb.htm

You can learn to deal with your symptoms, dis-ease and disease with tools that are introduced in this and other manuals, and explained in greater detail in *How Can I Heal What Hurts.* We can all learn to address our symptoms as challenges that invite us to discover more about ourselves. We then come away enriched through these self-healing exercises – rewarded by the clearing of our symptoms, but also rewarded even when our symptoms are not always eliminated. We can learn how to understand them and deal with them in new ways, and can learn to listen to what our inner self is inviting us to become aware of. This is also a road to spiritual awareness and spiritual healing.

Personal spirituality is the awareness of being part of something greater than our individual, physical selves. There is an enormous source of inspiration and healing available to us when we connect with our higher selves, with the energies that are a vital part of our inner and outer worlds, and with the world of spirits, nature spirits, angels and the Infinite Source.

If you are interested in learning about any of these ideas and approaches in greater depth, see the Suggested Reading List at the end of this manual.

**Suggestions:**

Write down problems in your life that you would like to address.

6

NOTES

Do you have any feelings of hurt, anger, fear, depression or any other feelings that bother you, which you would like to have less of?

Do you have negative beliefs about yourself or about others that get in your way of enjoying life? Write these down.

NOTES

did not feel safe expressing it, and found no other outlets for it. For years, I was easily angered by authority figures, particularly aggressive women.

As adults, we continue to stuff uncomfortable feelings inside, shutting a door behind them. Our unconscious resists releasing these emotions stuffed away in the caverns of our being – even when we are no longer in the painful situations that caused them; even when we are clearly in a better position to deal with them.

For instance, we might have buried anxieties and fears from when we were jealous of a younger or older brother or sister. As adults, if we encounter someone who is like our sister or brother, they may make us very uncomfortable – completely out of proportion to what is happening in the present; but we respond with unwarranted hurt or anger because the memories and feelings are stirred in the closets holding our feelings about our siblings. So, what do we do? We stuff more unpleasant feelings in our inner closets.

While self-healing techniques and various therapies can help to release some of these well-hidden traumas, our inner programs resist such efforts. Often, it is only when the emotional pus from past hurts festers to the point of serious physical and emotional pain that we even begin to become aware that something distressing is inside us.

## Suggestions:

Write down some of the childhood beliefs that persist from when you programmed them into your on-board computer. These are ideas that children often get when parents, teachers or other caregivers scold them or vent their angers on them.

For instance, do you say to yourself, "I'm [bad; dumb; stupid; clumsy; slow; ugly; or other negative characteristics] – things that might not be true?

# NOTES

Have you been told by others that you are too hard on your self or too self-critical? What are negative things you have said about yourself that others have questioned?

Write down ways of understanding the world that you have carried over from childhood – that look different from your view of yourself and the world today, and which you suspect might no longer be true, but which you don't see how you could change – but would like to change.

These often start with "I can't..." "I could never..."

For instance, do you believe:

I can't trust anybody because they'll just [cheat; hurt; take advantage of] me.

It's no use asking anyone to help me because people are just out to take care of themselves.

No one could like a person like me.

Write down the childhood beliefs you identify that get in the way of your enjoying life

# NOTES

## Taking responsibility for you issues: the first step towards dealing with problems

This workbook is designed to help you deal with your own problems and issues. It is all about how you can understand yourself better and change those aspects of your life that you are unhappy about. It is not about how to get other people to change, other than in ways that they may respond to you differently after you make changes in yourself.

### Suggestions:

Nobody can *make you* feel any emotion. How you respond to their behaviors is your choice. This may sound like a blaming statement, but it is not. Feeling sad, angry or hurt are natural ways to respond to unpleasant or hurtful experiences. Expecting others to change so that you will feel better is often not the best way to start feeling better. What they do will be their own choice. You have no control over them. What you can do, however, is to learn to understand your feelings and how to deal with them.

Return to page 5 and re-examine the issues you have listed that you would like to change. See how you can sharpen the focus of any of those statements about your life so that you take responsibility for your feelings, reactions to others and behaviors.

For instance, if any items on your list are about "She makes me so mad when…" or "He gets me all upset by…" then re-write these below, changing how you identify the problems. You might say, instead, "I get so mad when she…" or "I get all upset when he…"

# NOTES

## General ways to get ourselves out of trouble

*Things do not change; we change.*
– Thoreau

***Becoming aware*** that something is awry inside ourselves is the first step. We might wake up to this through feeling anxieties, fears, depression, anger or other emotions that appear to be stronger than we would expect in a given situation. We might develop pains, allergies or other physical symptoms that we and our doctors cannot explain according to conventional medical diagnoses. We may develop strains in our relationships that appear irrational. We may waken to inner turmoil through dreams and nightmares, or old memories of traumas may surface and surprise us.

***Embracing the problem*** is essential to dealing with it. Deepening our awareness of troublesome feelings, rather than running away from them or stuffing them back inside is essential. As adults we can develop better ways to deal with our feelings than through our child programs for avoiding them. This may be difficult to do at first, because it goes counter to a lifetime of running away and burying feelings.

***Developing self-healing methods to deal with problems*** allows us to lessen the intensity of negative feelings around them. Our feelings are what trap us in negative patterns.

***Developing positive attitudes and positive momentum*** in dealing with our problems makes it easier to deal with further problems. Success does breed success.

***Asking for help*** **to** deal with our problems makes a big difference. When we set our inner intention to get help; when we approach other people for help; and when we seek the help of a higher power we are inviting social, energetic, and spiritual supports that can help us to deal with our fears and hurts.

***Getting professional help*** can make a big difference. While our inner wisdom is aware of what is wrong with us, it may take us a long time to change our childhood programs and find the closets where the old hurts are buried, and another long time to release  what is in the closets.  A counselor, psychotherapist, spiritual healer or other complementary/ alternative therapy practitioner, or physician may be able to offer us shortcuts in this process of discovery and release.

# NOTES

***Volume I of Healing Research*** describes many ways in which spiritual healing can help; Volume II details how complementary therapies and bioenergy medicine can help. (See details under Recommended Reading at the end of this Manual.

***Feeling better about ourselves***, feeling more supported and more entitled to receive love and acceptance can help us address these feelings. This can come with time and maturity or with the support of family and friends.

***Building on progress and successes*** will help to consolidate your gains, provide satisfaction and encouragement to continue with the work of restructuring your beliefs and habits, and will build a 'feel-good' attitude towards working on yourself.

- Recording your successes in this workbook and in your personal journal can be a backbone to mapping your progress and your path forward.

- Sharing your progress with others in your family, circles of friends and colleagues will give you further feedback on the changes you are making, and the satisfaction of helping others to know they, too, can work on themselves to improve their lives on many levels.

- Attending in-person or telephone workshops with Dr. Benor can offer you a group of kindred spirits and explorers on similar paths with whom to share your progress, as well as your observations and suggestions regarding their progress, and from whom you can learn new and varied ways of using WHEE.

## Suggestions:

Write down the ways you deal with your problems that have helped, at least some of the time.

# NOTES

Write down suggestions you get from others for how to sharpen your understanding and use of WHEE.

# NOTES

Save this space for reminders to yourself of what parts of WHEE work best for you in dealing with various problems.

24

NOTES

## Principles for self-healing exercises

*Each difficult moment has the potential to open my eyes and open my heart.*

– Myla Kabat-Zinn

**Safety issues** come first. Do not do anything that is suggested in this manual, nor in any other setting, nor by any other authority if it does not feel right to you. There is no single way of helping or healing that works for everyone. If one method does not work for you, there will be others that will help.

Invite your unconscious mind and higher self to protect you when you start any journey of exploration. A simple affirmation or prayer can focus your mind and set the intent for safe healing.

Respect your own inner defenses. You developed these during times of stress, when these protected you from your anxieties, fears, pains and distress. Your unconscious mind, out of habit, believes that these defenses are still necessary. It is helpful to connect with your pains or other issues and dialogue with them, to be certain your inner self is ready to release them.

**Ground yourself regularly on waking in the morning and again before any activity that is important to you**. When we are on journeys of exploration in transpersonal/ spiritual dimensions we can easily lose touch with physical reality. Grounding ourselves by connecting with the earth and with our physical selves helps us maintain a healthy balance and helps to keep us from getting lost in spiritual dimensions – enabling us to draw nurturance from these dimensions in order to make our lives more balanced and whole. Breathing exercises, Yoga, t'ai chi, qigong, jogging, imagery meditations of linking with Gaia are some of the many ways to ground ourselves.

**Learn to connect with your intuition**. This involves pattern recognition, body-mind connections, psychic awareness and transpersonal/spiritual awareness. Intuition will help you to uncover issues that your unconscious mind is inviting you to address, to screen methods that can help you, and to assess your progress. Again, there is no single method that will work for everyone. Explore a variety of ways to access your intuition so that if one does not work, you will have others to use. You may also find that different methods work better in different situations.

# NOTES

***Connect with your inner self and with others through your heart***. We may be stressed over not understanding why we feel a certain way or over not knowing what to do about problems. These are questions posed by the head. They may have multiple answers or no clear answers at present – in either case leaving us without a clear basis for responding to challenges. When we cannot reason our way through a problem, it is often the *feelings* we have *about* the situation which are the problem.

Responses from the head tend to come from sets of expectations and rules, imposing structure on our perceptions, our interpretations of situations and our responses. Responses from the heart come from a more open, healing place – where every experience may be an invitation to become more heart centered, responding with compassion, love and healing rather than with logical and reasoned responses.

***Make one small change at a time in your personal practice or in the focus of the healing and observe the differences in your responses***. This will provide helpful feedback in navigating your way through new and unfamiliar territories of your consciousness and of transpersonal dimensions.

***Write down exactly what you say when you use affirmations***. The unconscious mind is extremely concrete and literal. It responds precisely to the words you use, very much like a computer. If it is not responding the way you expect or wish it to, it may help to re-examine the words you have spoken to phrase the problem and to express your feelings. Sometimes a little shift or tweak to the wording will produce a major difference in your response to WHEE and to other self-healing methods that rely on affirmations. Similarly, if you are interrupted in your work, it is helpful to have the exact words you were using when you return to the healing.

***Journal your progress***. Writing down your experiences, thoughts, feelings, dreams and inner explorations in a personal journal helps to keep your focus. It also provides a diary of your progress, which can be helpful in your growth. Make an appointment with yourself at regular intervals to note your progress – your changes and growth – through using WHEE.

***Be patient and gentle with yourself*** as you explore and learn new approaches and move deeper in your awareness. Do not compare yourself with others who may be working on different issues at different rates of progress. Each of us is a unique individual with our own issues and challenges and with our own ways of sorting these out.

28

NOTES

*Find teachers of integrity whom you respect and admire* and ask as many questions as you need to ask in order to learn what you want and need to learn. Teachers may have wisdom to share that is part of the lessons they are still learning. Remember that the teaching and the teacher may not be one and the same, although the lessons are better when this congruence is present.

*Ask and pray for what you feel will be for your highest good and for the highest good of all.*

**Suggestions:**

Write down ways in which you notice your intuition is working.

Write several ways you will use to ground yourself regularly, every day, and also when you feel stressed.

Write some times down here and in your diary when you will do the grounding exercises.

Remember to connect with others through your heart.

Write in your journal daily.

# NOTES

# WHEE

## Safety issues

*An affirmation for safety* is a protection as you work on your issues. You will want to develop your own phrases that feel and work best for you, but here are several generic affirmations as starters, which I have found useful for myself and others whom I have helped.

"I accept only that which is for my highest good."

"I ask [God; my higher self; Christ; my guardian angels] to protect me as I do this work."

"May God, who made me, make me well, as I am meant to be."

## Suggestions:

Write several affirmations for safety that feel helpful to you.

Ask others what affirmations have been helpful to them and write down any that you feel may work well for you.

# NOTES

***Ask your symptoms [pain, anxiety, fears, etc.] whether they are ready to be released.*** If you get a 'yes,' then before you start to work on releasing them, ask your symptoms why they have been there, how they developed over the time they were there, and what they want to tell you.

Write down all of the answers you get.

*Example 1 (Examples use assumed names, composite cases):*

> 'Greta' suffered from terrible stomachaches, which had been present most of her life. Numerous visits to many doctors and complementary therapists and numerous medications and remedies had produced only minimal, transient relief. The question to her stomachaches, "What do you want to tell me?" had never been asked. Greta was astounded to have the clear, distinct answer appear in her mind – that she was swallowing down her angers, and had been doing this since childhood. Her stomach was speaking for her inner self, wanting her to find a better way to handle her angers.
>
> This inner dialogue was the start of her self-healing for her stomachaches. Greta used WHEE on her angers, both past and current, to deal with them in a healthier way. Her stomachaches cleared in a few weeks.

If you get a 'no' about whether you are ready to release your symptoms, it is likewise helpful to ask them, "Why are you here?" and "In what ways are you helping me?" and "What would it take for you to leave?"

Symptoms take on lives of their own. Respect your inner defenses. You developed these during times of stress, when these protected you from your anxieties, fears, pains and distress. Your unconscious mind, out of habit, believes these defenses are still needed. If your symptoms do not trust it is safe or in your best interests to leave, you can ask them to explain why they feel you still need them. If you are unable to convince them to leave, you can still ask, "Can I let go of *some parts* of these symptoms?"

# NOTES

**Suggestions:**

Write down symptoms you have, such as pains or anger responses, and ask yourself, "What are ways that these may have helped me in my life?" (In the past; in the present.)

As much as a pain is something you suffer from, what are ways in which the pain has become a familiar friend or a helper?

List any ways in which your symptom may help you not have to do something you'd rather not do.

List ways in which your pain may give you permission to ask others to help you more than you might otherwise request their assistance.

# NOTES

## Grounding and centering before starting to use WHEE

Any of the following methods can help you to release distracting thoughts and feelings, connect with the center of your being where peace and wisdom reside, and get yourself into a frame of mind and state of being that are conducive to doing serious inner work.

**Breathe deeply several times**, picturing to yourself that you are releasing tensions and inhaling healing energies.

**Sit quietly and sense that you have energy roots going deep into the earth**, through which you can draw in calming, healing energies. At the same time, you can release any negative energies through these roots, deep into the earth. The earth is an excellent composter, and can transmute the negative energies into energetic fertilizer. You might also synchronize this imagery with your breathing.

**Brain balancing exercises** ('Brain Gym') can quickly balance your energies and harmonize right and left brain hemispheres.

- *Lazy eights* – Trace a large figure eight that is lying on its side, using the thumb of one hand at arm's length in front of you and reaching as far right and left as your arm will extend. Let your eyes follow your thumb, without moving your head. After you have traced three eights in the air, reverse the direction of tracing the figure eight, doing it in this direction for three times. Repeat this with your left hand; then with both hands.

- *Practice cross-crawl motions* – While standing, rhythmically raise your left knee and move the elbow of your right arm towards the left knee, touching elbow to knee if you can; alternate this with raising your right knee, moving your left elbow towards that knee. Do this six times to each side.

**Breathing awareness** can be a quick way to ground yourself. Take three slow, deep breaths, being aware of the air and the energies it brings you as it enters your lungs.

If you have more time for grounding, this can be turned into a meditation. Simply watch your breath coming in and out, acknowledging your inhalation silently with the word, 'in' and exhalation with the word, 'out.' If any thoughts, feelings, or sensory stimulation come along to distract you, gently return your focus to your breathing – noting to yourself that you can give the distraction your full attention after you are through meditating.

# NOTES

**Suggestions:**

Take one of the above at a time, practicing it several times daily for a week. Note here or in your journal how you feel after doing this. You may notice progressive change that encourage you to continue any one or several of these for more than a week.

Write down which of these, or other grounding exercises you may find elsewhere, are most helpful.

# NOTES

***Setting your intent can strengthen the effects of WHEE.*** Once you are comfortable doing these brain balancing exercises, you can also use them to set your intent for success with WHEE. State an affirmation to yourself, prior to starting these movements. For example, I will:

be clear and focused in working on my issues;

connect always from my heart with those in my life;

remember to ____;
  ask for my needs to be met, trusting that the universe/ God/ Infinite Source/ my community of family and friends will respond;

____ Pick one of your own...

Then do the brain balancing exercises. I have been impressed, both in my personal practice and in counseling others, how this setting of intent can promote and facilitate progress within ourselves, interpersonally and transpersonally. My thanks to Martina Steiger for introducing this to me.

## Suggestions:

Write helpful intentions of your own as these occur to you

# NOTES

Take one intent from your list, state if firmly before doing your grounding exercises. Do this regularly for a week with this one intent. Note how helpful (or not) this has been for you before you start on the next intent.

Note which grounding exercise seems to work the best for you with your intents.

# NOTES

## Background of WHEE

When I learned about psychotherapy as a teenager, I knew that was what I wanted to do. I couldn't imagine anyone actually getting paid to do something so fascinating. I studied psychology as my undergraduate pre-med major, endured the challenges of medical school, with a year's break for a National Institute of Mental Health research fellowship in psychiatry and for regrouping my battered energies. I trained as a psychiatrist 1967-1973, (with two intervening years in the US Air Force during the Vietnam War), when psychiatry was mostly psychotherapy. Over the years, managed care has squeezed psychiatrist towards medication management. While I've resisted prescribing medications exclusively, it is pretty difficult to do much psychotherapy in a 15-20 minute medication visit – the length of time allowed under managed care.

Fortunately, I worked mostly with children (in a clinic and a day hospital), and was allowed the 'luxury' of 30-minute sessions because I had to speak with parents, teachers, school counselors, and pediatricians, in addition to pharmacists and managed care companies -- all in addition to speaking with the children.

I constantly sought to develop ways of providing psychotherapy along with the medications, but was unable within my limited timeframe to use the psychodynamic approaches I was taught as a psychiatric resident. Eye Movement Desensitization and Reprocessing (EMDR) was a blessing to me, as well as to my clients. I was able to use EMDR with children who had post-traumatic stress disorders, as children respond very quickly to this approach – not having barnacles on their problems like adults do. I also used EMDR to de-stress myself.

With adults, it is recommended that EMDR should be done only during sessions with the therapist. This is to prevent being overwhelmed by intense emotional releases that can occur during treatment. I found that children rarely had such intense releases, perhaps because they had not kept their hurt feelings bottled up for as long a time, or perhaps because their emotional defenses are not a strongly developed. Another factor may be that I am comfortable doing this, having used EMDR for myself without the constant guidance of a therapist.

Since I usually see children with their parents, I also taught the more stable parents to guide their children in using the EMDR at home. If the children were mature and responsible, I encouraged them to practice the eye movements on their own – at home or at school, whenever they were upset.

# NOTES

This was very helpful, for instance, for children who had post-traumatic stress disorder (PTSD) with nightmares, when traumatic memories were stimulated by current stresses, or where excessive angers erupted. I still worried, however, that there might be intense emotional releases which could be traumatic.

I then learned to use the Emotional Freedom Technique (EFT) of Gary Craig, and other Meridian Based Therapy (MBT) approaches. In EFT and its related therapies you tap or press a finger at a series of acupuncture points on your face, chest and hand, while reciting an affirmation. (Affirmations are described below.) Because it works more rapidly than EMDR and does not evoke intense emotional releases, it can be used as self-healing.

This works more quickly than EMDR, with extra advantages. Because it works rapidly and does not evoke intense emotional releases, I offer "two (or three) for the price of one" introductions to EFT to children together with their mothers; including their fathers as well when they are present. This way, the children more often accept the therapy and comply with the recommendation to use WHEE at home to deal with stresses. Parents are more confident it will work because they have experienced its benefits themselves, and therefore encourage their children to use it more often.

I had difficulty introducing EFT in my work settings. EMDR has an extensive research base to confirm its efficacy in treating post-traumatic stress disorders (PTSDs). On the basis of my certification in EMDR, I was able to obtain official permission (from the administrators of the child and adolescent clinic where I work) to use this with their clients. (See Research references at the end of the manual.) Because EFT has no research base, they would not grant me permission to use it. Giving this a hard think, I turned it around and now call it an 'affirmation technique.' No one has faulted me for using affirmations in therapy, and never mind what clients do with their hands on their own bodies while they recite these.

In an introductory workshop by Asha Nahoma Clinton on *Matrix Therapy*, Asha suggested that alternating tapping the eyebrow points while reciting the affirmation works just as well as the entire series of EFT points. Ever conscious of my time limitations, I immediately started exploring this hybrid approach, that combines aspects of EMDR and EFT (which I now call the Wholistic Hybrid derived from EMDR and EFT, or WHEE).

I address each of the components of WHEE separately, although they are clearly a unified process for self-healing.

# NOTES

## Right and left stimulation

EMDR was born when Francine Shapiro, a California psychologist, noticed that feelings of depression lifted when she spontaneously started moving her eyes back and forth, right and left. She developed this as the basis of her treatment. Initially, the therapist guided the client in these rhythmic movements of their eyes from right to left and back. Needless to say, this could become a tiring process! A horizontal bar with a row of LED lights automated the guidance of eye movements back and forth. However, some people could not tolerate this because they developed vertigo or nausea.

Auditory stimulation alternating to right and left ears solved much of these problems, and again, automated systems were developed to relieve therapists of the chore of rubbing their fingers next to clients' ears for this mode of right and left stimulation.

It was then discovered that right and left kinesthetic stimulation will work as well. Clients can tap or pat their right and left thigh, or alternate tapping their feet on the floor. Alternating tapping on the end of the eyebrow that is closest to the nose on the right and left sides nearest to the nose has the extra advantage that these are acupressure releasing points. Another variation is the 'butterfly hug.' This is the self-treatment intervention that is most popular in my clinical experience, particularly with children: clients' arms are crossed so that each hand rests on the opposite biceps muscles of the arm, and they alternate patting on each arm with their hands. Many find the self-hug comforting, in addition to being highly effective in combination with the affirmation.

You may find that touching your body lightly works best, or a firmer tap or pat my feel better. Similarly, the rate of tapping can be as fast or as slow as you find comfortable.

Teenagers would often refuse to use any of these tapping approaches outside of the therapy room. Their typical comment was, "Sure, Dad! Like I'm going to tap my forehead or pat my arms in front of my friends! They'll think I'm some sort of nut case!" I speculated to myself that if they alternated tapping with their tongue on their teeth on the left and then on the teeth on the right this should work just as well, and found that indeed it does. Another private possibility is to alternate tightening the toes of the feet so that no one can see the right and left stimulation. These approaches have been received much better by those who are shy or uncomfortable with tapping in public. Whichever works best for you is the approach you should use.

# NOTES

*Example 2:*

> *'Sol,' a ten year-old fourth grader, found WHEE helpful in dealing with his severe school phobia. The method that worked best for him was tapping his eyebrow points. He was embarrassed to do this in front of his classmates. We arranged with his teacher that he could excuse himself to the restroom, where he would sit in a toilet stall and do his tapping behind the closed door.*

Working on your issues when you are not stressed is highly recommended before you work on them in stressful situations. You wouldn't expect to go out on a sports field for a serious game without practicing beforehand. It is the same with using WHEE in serious situations. Sol practiced using WHEE on his fears of going to school for several days at home before he used WHEE in school.

In some cases, the original method of moving your eyes rhythmically back and forth, from right to left and back, may work better. Some people find that this causes slight dizziness or nausea.

A deep breath following the affirmation facilitates releases and can enhance the effects of the process. Similarly, holding your other hand over your heart center (chakra) while you tap or touch your eyebrow points deepens the effects.

## Suggestions:

Keep a log on this page and/or in your journal of issues that you work on, which forms of right and left stimulation you used, and which form worked best for that issue. Over a period of time you may find that one form generally works best for most or all of your problems, or you may note that for some issues there is one form of stimulation that is better, while for other issues another form works better.

52

NOTES

## Affirmations

Here is a generic affirmation adapted from EFT:

> Even though I have this [anxiety, panic, fear, etc. – be specific when filling in the blank],
> I wholly and completely love and accept myself,
> and God loves and accepts me wholly and completely and unconditionally.
> (Use whatever strong positive statement suits you best at the time you need it.)

It is very helpful to write down the precise words you use in stating your affirmation. The unconscious mind is extremely literal and concrete. It may respond one way to "I feel distressed when I think of _____" and very differently to "I feel [angry; furious; hurt] when I think of _____." When you have written down the words you are using, you can go back and tweak the affirmation if it is not working well. Conversely, if you get interrupted, you can return and see the words that were working marvelously well for you.

Keeping these notes in a notebook or journal can be a help to you in other ways, as discussed below.

Younger children use simpler affirmations, such as: "Even though I feel ____ when I think about ____, I love myself a lot."

None of these affirmations is meant to be written in stone. They are simply suggestions of strong positive statements that we can use to follow the framing of the problems we are addressing. People who don't feel they can say, "I love and accept myself," or "God loves and accepts me" can say, "I remember a time when I was [calm/ happy/ joyful/ at peace];" "I know [my mother/ father/ spouse/ pet] [loves me; is there for me]." A little boy who had been horribly abused used the following, which for him was a strong positive affirmation: "At least now I'm safe and my father can't beat me any more."

## Suggestion:

Write down several strong positive affirmations that feel good to you.

# NOTES

## Assessing progress

**The SUDS:** Prior to using WHEE, it is helpful to assess how strong the negative feeling is that you want to address. The most commonly used method is the *Subjective Units of Distress Scale* (SUDS), where you rate discomfort/ distress on a scale from 0 (not bothering you at all) to 10 (the worst it could possibly feel).

After tapping for a few minutes, check the SUDS again. It will usually go down. Repeat the assessing and tapping until it is zero. Then you can build up a positive affirmation to replace the negative, simply stating the positive as you tap.

If the numbers do not shift after you tap a round of WHEE, you can give yourself a gentle massage on the *releasing spot*, located just below the collar bone at its midpoint. No affirmation is needed here. Then return to tapping.

**Body feedback for progress:** As you connect initially with the negative issues you want to release, notice any sensations in your body. Commonly, we may feel tension in our chest, stomach, jaws, neck or back; pains; tightness when we breathe; or other symptoms. Any and all of these can serve as markers for being 'up tight' as you start to work on your issues, with lessening of body sensations as you release the issues.

## Suggestions:

If you have not been used to checking how strongly you feel about issues in your life, then ask yourself whenever you notice yourself responding with feeling to a situation, "How strong is my feeling right now, on the scale of '1' to '10' ?" Record notable information you get through checking in this way.

# NOTES

Here is an invitation to be a detective: See whether you have patterns of 'bodyspeak' of these sorts. For instance, do you get headaches on Sunday evening or Monday morning that might be speaking to your about issues that make you tense in your job or studies? Do such symptoms occur when you are around particular people? After eating certain foods?

Invite your body to speak to you in words or images when you have symptoms – especially when they are recurring ones. Write down your observations here.

# NOTES

If you have a tension, tightness, ache or other sensation in your body, ask your body, "What are you wanting me to pay attention to in my life right now?" Write down some of the information your body has given you. This might have to do with diet, exercise, posture, rest or other issues. Write down what you learn your body wants in the left column. It is surprising how easily we can forget messages of this sort when we are not used to listening to our inner self in these ways. See how this inner witness helps you in your detective work.

_____|_____

_____|_____

_____|_____

_____|_____

_____|_____

_____|_____

_____|_____

_____|_____

_____|_____

_____|_____

_____|_____

_____|_____

Next, go back and write down in the right column what you promise your body you will do to meet its needs. Again, it is helpful to review this 'promises' page regularly, even every day, as it may be challenging to remember and follow through on your promises.

# NOTES

## Learning with incremental, step by step changes

***Make one small change at a time in your personal practice or in the focus of the WHEE and then observe the difference in your responses.*** This will provide helpful feedback in navigating your way through new and unfamiliar territories of your consciousness and of transpersonal dimensions.

For instance, you will want to check out which of the various ways of right and left brain stimulation work best for you. While the most popular, especially with children, tends to be the butterfly hug, this is a very individual matter and you may find that tapping your eyebrows or scrunching up your toes works best for you. Be aware that different tapping approaches may work better for different issues or at different times.

Tweaking your affirmations may make a big difference in your progress with a specific issue. Having the input of someone you trust, either a family member, friend, or therapist may be helpful in developing new variations on familiar ways that you phrase issues, in looking at related issues that may be blocking your progress (but may not be obvious to you because you cannot see the trees for the forest of issues in which you are lost), or in identifying meta-issues (see below) that are blocking releases and creating resistance.

### Suggestion:

Even if you have been doing perfectly well with a particular statement of a problem or of an affirmation, tweak it a little just to get a sense of how your responses change as you change what you are saying or doing.

Write down here or in your journal some of the different changes you experience in response to shifts and tweaks in your statements of problems and affirmations.

When you find a phrase that works particularly well, put a star next to it so that you can use is as an example for further helpful phrasing in new statements of problems and affirmations.

# NOTES

## Dealing with resistances

If the number does not change after a round of WHEE, this is called 'resistance.' First check to be certain you have focused your affirmation in the best way possible. When this does not overcome the block, resistance is effectively managed in most cases by massaging the sore-spot/ releasing point below the midpoint of the collar bone. Then return to using WHEE and the affirmation. If this does not produce results, tweak the affirmation to see whether you are truly on target with the issues that are being addressed.

You may want to vary the ways in which you are stimulating your right and left brain. As noted above, different tapping approaches may work better for different issues or at different times.

You may find it helpful to use muscle testing (described below) to ask questions such as: "Am I ready to release some of this distress?" "Is there some part of me that wants to hold onto some of this issue, or to some of the ways I deal with this issue?" Again, you may need to tweak the question in order to get a helpful answer.

The brain balancing exercises (p. 37) may clear resistances.

If the above techniques and dialoguing with your symptoms do not clear up the resistance issues, you may want to consult a therapist who can help you explore and address your resistances.

64

NOTES

## Installing positives to replace negatives that have been released

If you stop working with WHEE on an issue after it has been brought to a zero, there is a distinct possibility that some of the negative feelings could return, though rarely to the level of their initial intensity. To a great degree such recurrences are simply a matter of habit, often stimulated by being in situations or relationships that bring back the old memories and feelings associated with the issue.

To prevent recurrence of the released issues, you can install positives that replace the negatives. You do this by starting with a statement that in some way is an opposite to the released issue. You assess the SUDS for the positive (0 = I hardly feel/believe this at all to 10 = this is the strongest it can be), then recite the positive statement, followed by the positive affirmation – while tapping in whatever way feels the best to you. After each round of tapping, you pause and assess the SUDS. In doing the positive portion of WHEE you will find the numbers getting stronger.

As with resistance in doing the WHEE for negatives, if the SUDS does not change for the positive, massage the releasing point and return to tapping.

When working on difficult traumas, be patient with yourself in sorting out a positive statement. It can be challenging to develop positives when you are dealing with a serious accident, loss of someone dear to you, or a rape.

*Example 3:*

> *Working on his chronic headaches on his own, at home, 'Mike' assessed his SUDS and said, "Even though I have this vice-like pain in my temples, I wholly and completely love and accept myself, and God loves and accepts me wholly and completely and unconditionally." He worked on this until his SUDS came down to zero.*
>
> *He then decided his positive would be: "I can be in stressful situations and not get a headache, and I wholly and completely love and accept myself, and God loves and accepts me wholly and completely and unconditionally." He found that the SUDS did not go up, even when he massaged the releasing spot. I reviewed the affirmation with him and he tweaked it to say, "I can be in stressful situations and remain calm and relaxed, and…" This worked immediately and he brought it up to a '10' after 6 rounds of WHEE.*

# NOTES

Note that Mike stated his successful positive in positive language. He did not use phrases such as: "I *won't* get headaches" or "I'm *not* going to worry about getting another headache." The unconscious mind does not deal well with negatives, and often tends to latch onto the statement of the emotions. In the above examples of what not to say, the unconscious mind would be likely register: "I get headaches" and "I'm going to worry about getting another headache."

*Example 4:*

> *Six-year old 'Sally' had been neglected and abused emotionally, physically and sexually by her father from at least the age of two and probably earlier. She had also witnessed violence between her parents. She was removed from her home at age four, and was re-traumatized in a series of foster home placements – where the welfare worker did not tell the foster parents to expect irritability, temper outbursts, sleep onset delays till early hours of the morning, night terrors, and bedwetting. Her then current foster mother requested that Sally have counseling when her teacher repeatedly called the foster mother to take her home from school for disrespecting the teacher and hitting other children.*

> *I was immediately impressed with her inability to sit still, high levels of impulsivity and distractibility, difficulty attending to and misunderstanding questions I asked, along with a history of forgetfulness and disorganization. I diagnosed PTSD and possible attention deficit hyperactivity disorder (ADHD). I prescribed small doses of Ritalin. Despite public controversy over this medication, I find it one of the more gentle and helpful of the prescriptions I write. Its effects are evident within minutes if the dose is right. If effective, I felt that this could provide rapid relief for some of Sally's problems. She responded well to the medication and within two days was the teacher was pleased to report she could sit still and attend in class, was less impulsive, less forgetful and no longer had temper outbursts. However, her difficulties settling and sleeping at night persisted. We also arranged for counseling sessions weekly with a psychologist, focused on issues of adjusting to her new family, multiple losses (parental and foster families), and PTSD issues.*

> *At the initial interview, I taught Sally and her foster mother WHEE, using the butterfly hug. Sally liked the exercise, finding the butterfly hug comforting, in and of itself. For her first round, she chose to work on one of the recurrent nightmares she had of being chased by a*

# NOTES

*monster with big teeth who wanted to bite he. She was unable to count, so I had her show me with the gap between her hands how big her bad feeling was when she thought about the monster chasing her in her nightmare. She opened her arms wide and said, "I can't reach to show you how big the scary feeling is." Within minutes of using the butterfly hug and reciting the WHEE affirmation for children, her hands were touching each other when I asked her to show me how bad it felt. She had reduced the scary feelings to zero.*

*Over the next several weeks, Sally (with the help of her foster mother) used the butterfly hug daily on her many fears, difficulty falling asleep, and nightmares, as well as to calm down after she had angry outbursts.*

*Within two months, Sally was functioning at near-normal levels of behavior in school and at home. Counseling continued weekly for another six months and was then tapered and stopped. I have followed her for Ritalin prescriptions for three years and we have all been pleased with her excellent academic progress and with her good behavioral and social adjustments in school and at home.*

## Suggestions:

Write down a variety of positives that you would like to use to replace some of the challenges in your life that you wrote down on page 5. Make sure you use positive language, avoiding phrases such as, "I won't…" or "I am not…"

# NOTES

## Cognitive restructuring with WHEE

*Insanity is doing the same thing over and over again and expecting different results.*
– Albert Einstein

**WHEE helps us to shift our limiting beliefs and disbeliefs**, such as "I could never [succeed at ___; talk in public; handle my mother-in-law, boss or abusive partner]" or "I don't deserve to [be loved; enjoy myself; succeed]" or "I am [bad; stupid; ugly]." In these instances we use the SUDS to assess how strongly we feel these beliefs or disbeliefs are true, and then proceed to use WHEE in the same way as deal with emotional issues – reducing the negatives and installing positives.

**WHEE helps us to address problems with appropriate concern, without the added layers of worry** that we often add to our concerns. Concern is the logical, 'Mr. Spock' (of Star Treck) way; the 'Adult' (of Transactional Analysis) way of dealing with issues. We ask, "What is the challenge?" and sort out the logical ways to deal with it, accepting that in a less than perfect world we can only do the best we can. Worry is the overlay of meta-anxieties about how we are managing to deal with these issues; the "Oh, my goodness! I don't know how I'm going to handle this!" or the "This is too much to bear, on top of all of the other problems I have to deal with!"

**WHEE enables us to release the worries, installing positive attitudes and focus** to replace those wheel-spinning wastes of our time – that are born out of childhood programs. We can then use our maximal energies to address the concerns.

## Suggestions:

Write down several beliefs or disbeliefs about yourself that you would like to change.

# NOTES

Write several ways of stating the opposite of each belief, in preparation for installing this positive after you have dealt with the problem belief.

Write down several issues you tend to worry about. Consider whether you would prefer to change these worries into concerns, and if so, what affirmations would help you to do so.

# NOTES

## Partializing problems

***Addressing a piece of a problem at a time allows us to manage small bites with WHEE*** so that we aren't stuck with affirmations and issues we cannot digest in one round of WHEE. By breaking a problem into its component parts and issues, we can address each one on its own.

*Example 5.*

> *Sam was struggling with his job as a bottom-level manager in a large appliance firm. He was a proud and for the most part happy husband and father to two young children. He came for help with WHEE because he had a weight problem that he constantly worried and fretted about, feeling that he was unattractive and therefore making a poor impression at work and unable to achieve his full potential professionally. He was also worried that his wife might be finding him unattractive, because his sexual relationship with his wife was becoming less and less satisfying.*
>
> *Sam's obesity had resisted all previous therapies. His self-esteem was obviously low because of his weight. We explored his history carefully, clarifying that he had started to gain weight at age eight, after his mother died in an accident. He missed her deeply, and was unable to express his grief because his father had told him to "Be strong!" and "Don't be a cry-baby." Sam realized that he had started comfort eating to fill the void of his missing mother.*
>
> *Over the years, Sam's self-image became an issue because of the obesity. Children teased him about his looks and when he was unable to keep up in athletics with others who were more physically fit. His comfort eating, that had gotten him into this problem, was no help in coping with these secondary stresses that resulted from his obesity. Though he struggled to stick with the diets that his family doctor and school nurse recommended, and that his father pestered him to watch, he could not overcome his comfort eating habits. Now, as an adult, he hesitated to stand up and speak in public because he was so self-conscious about his weight. His wife reminded him frequently not to snack. Sam took these expressions of her concern as criticisms and was increasingly cross and irritable with her, which was putting a strain on their relationship.*
>
> *Sam was motivated to work hard to sort out his eating and self-image*

# NOTES

*issues. He diligently outlined all of the issues that appeared to be related to his obesity, such as:*

> *- particular snack foods he liked and craved*

> *- stresses that he handled by eating*

> *- negative things he tended to say about his body*

> *- negative things he said to himself about failing to stick to a diet and lose weight*

> *- things he did not do because he was embarrassed to stand up in front of people*

*Sam was pleased to find that WHEE gave him a tool with which he could address any issue he chose to address. Some problems, like his cravings for specific foods, responded rapidly. Others, such as his self-criticisms and his embarrassment over his looks, were more difficult and took longer to resolve. Working on one issue at a time gave Sam a growing sense of success and achievement, which encouraged him to work that much harder and enabled him to tolerate distress better. For instance, he was able to release many years' accumulations of hurts and angers over people teasing him, so that he no longer took his wife's concern as a dig at his being overweight. In other words, he developed a sweetening spiral. With more self-confidence, he took more risks and had more successes at work.*

Partializing enabled Sam to change his long-time, frustrating problem that had resisted treatment into a series of smaller issues that he could readily address with WHEE.

Partializing may help us identify a block to our progress, where we may be willing and ready to release certain parts of our problem but may have one or more issues that keep us from releasing the entire bundle. Partializing also allows us to follow the threads of individual issues that my lead in different directions. (See also discussion on *bundling*, below, the opposite of partializing.)

> *The smallest change in perspective can transform a life.*
> *What tiny attitude adjustment might turn your world around?*
> – Oprah

# NOTES

## Suggestions:

Write down several knotty problems. Next to each, write out the component parts that you might address separately.

# NOTES

## Meta-emotions and meta-beliefs

It is common to experience anxiety or other feelings about the process of letting go of habitual ways of dealing with feelings and beliefs. Common meta-worries are: "If I let this out it will hurt too much for me to bear!" or "I could never [handle; succeed; be accepted if I let out these feelings]…" or "If I open the lid on this bucket of stuffed feelings, it will smell so bad that no one will be willing to deal with me any more."

Meta-emotions and beliefs can block us from releasing buried feelings and memories. As discussed above, at the time when we buried them, often in childhood or when we were under severe stress, we were in positions where they could have been experienced as overwhelming. At those times it was adaptive to bury them outside our conscious awareness in order to prevent or at least diminish our suffering.

Keeping away from the buried feelings becomes a habit, reinforced for months and years by fears of the unconscious mind about releasing the buried feelings. When we use WHEE to release the old feelings from the closets and caves where they were carefully locked away, the unconscious mind may become anxious. We are telling the unconscious mind to switch gears and change its habits – programs that have protected us, by its childish understanding, from the pain of experiencing these buried feelings.

We may therefore have to use WHEE on the meta-beliefs and emotions in order to release the habitual locks on the doors of the closets wherein lie the skeletons of old traumas. Once past these locks, we can then address the feelings themselves.

*Example 6:*

> *I used WHEE to clear some of my own childhood fears of abandonment, stimulated by moving to a new home abroad at age four and never again seeing the nanny who had been with me from the earliest months of my life; later moving back to the US at age eight when my parents separated and, in effect, losing my father then. For several rounds of WHEE this was going well, with my SUDS dropping from a '9' to a '6.' Then I hit resistance that was not relieved by massaging the releasing spot, nor by tweaking my affirmations. The SUDS simply would not budge. Looking for reasons for the block to progress, I uncovered a fear that if I were to open the door to the closet where those old feelings were safely locked away, they would be more than I could handle. The*

# NOTES

*words that came to me were, "there would be no one there to pick me up if I fell."*

*Sensing this was a meta-block causing the resistance, I used WHEE on that phrase. This released the block and I was able to work through my feelings about the abandonments.*

*That phrase, however, was also a doorway into another closet with buried memories. At age three I had slipped on the top rung of a playground slide, falling and fracturing my ankle. This occurred when I was visiting with friends of my mother, when she was attending school. I uncovered a distinct memory that at the time I slipped, I realized that for some reason I had actually let myself slip. In other words, this apparent accident was contrived by my unconscious mind, seeking attention I felt was sorely missing in my life – my mother being unavailable because of her studies and my father being unavailable, living in another country. Contrary to my hopes in my childhood contrivance to get more attention, I actually got less – as I was unable to play with the other children and was left alone with various toys, which soon became boring.  Here, too, WHEE was helpful in releasing the old hurts.*

It is not at all uncommon to find layers upon layers of buried hurts like these. I have come to call this, "Peeling the never-ending onion of life."

**Suggestions:**

Write down any meta-emotions you may notice, in response to the emotions you experience when you get upset.

Write down affirmations you can use to release these meta-emotions.

# NOTES

## Dealing with insufficient motivation to change

Motivation can be addressed with WHEE just like any other issue. It is often sufficient to simply use the affirmation, "My motivation is strong and firm."

Blocks to motivation can be addressed and diminished.

For instance:

Even though I lack the motivation to...

Even though I procrastinate in...

Even though some part of me doesn't want to...

Even though my head says yes but my inner child is screaming, "No! Don't' go there!"...

## Suggestions:

Write down any resistances you feel about your willingness and intent to start and to persist in dealing with your issues.

Write down affirmations you can use to change these blocks to changing.

# NOTES

## Choosing a focus for WHEE

People commonly ask,

> "I've got a lifetime's accumulation of cobwebs. What corners do I clear first?"

> "Where should I start with this vacuum cleaner called WHEE?" "Should I dab a little WHEE on some of the scrapes, or should I use WHEE for major reconstructive surgery?"

If there is a therapist present to guide and direct the process, I suggest that it is best to start with the very worst fear or hurt. WHEE can help with any and every sort of problem. Once a person experiences the relief of WHEE for the more severe issues, s/he will be able to approach any other problem with confidence that it will respond.

If a therapist is not present for individual attention, as in workshops where there are many participants, or in the telephone tutorials I offer, then it is better not to begin with the worst possible issues; rather to start on an issue that has a SUDS intensity of 5 or greater, so that there is plenty of room to experience the success of WHEE, but not the liability of getting caught addressing a problem that rouses meta-anxieties which the person may not feel competent to handle.

*Example 7:*

> *In a one-hour workshop I did at a mental health center, a young woman volunteered as the subject for a demonstration of WHEE. She indicated that she had a severe issue of hurt and betrayal she wanted to work on. My intuition said, "Go for it!" though my logical mind was raising all sorts of alarms about "What if's" such as "What will you do if this woman stops in the middle because she's embarrassed to continue in front of the audience, and ends up with her hurts stuck in her throat?" and "How will it look if this woman falls apart in front of her colleagues?" I listened to my intuition, which was indicating a clear and strong 'yes.' We went for it.*

*I asked 'Bella' to name the feelings surrounding the issue, and she said, "hurt, betrayal and fear." She was not comfortable revealing the specific circumstances of her trauma, which had occurred in childhood. She used*

# NOTES

*WHEE tapping her eyebrows and with the butterfly hug but her SUDS didn't budge from 10, even after rubbing the releasing point under her collarbone.*

*I was beginning to sweat a little, but continued, asking Bella whether she felt it was safe to release these feelings. She responded with a strong "No." Considering that her trauma had occurred many years earlier, and that she was no longer in danger from the same situation, she readily agreed to address her meta-anxieties, which were at a SUDS of 9. These came down to zero in two rounds of WHEE with the butterfly hug.*

*Bella then felt she could work on the trauma. To her surprise (and mine!), her SUDS went all the way down to zero in one round of WHEE. She was silent for several minutes, obviously very moved by this experience. I asked whether she was ok, and she responded with a deep feeling of gratitude to God for having brought her to this point of release and forgiveness.*

*Bella explained to her colleagues that this was the most profound personal spiritual experience she had ever had.*

I have had only a few people respond as quickly and deeply and profoundly as Bella did. I more commonly see the SUDS shifting in jumps of three to five numbers in a single round of WHEE.

## Suggestions:

Explore whether a light focus or a more substantial one feels better to you with any given issue. With experience, many people find that they are able to clear much more of their issues, more quickly, if they address major aspects of an issue. When they do this, the minor issues are also cleared. Others find that dismantling and remodeling the structure of their issues and defenses one room or even one brick at a time works better. It's a little like the difference between going into a cold swimming pool one toe at a time or jumping in. There is best overall way. There is only what works best for you.

After using WHEE for a while, you might go back and review issues you have worked on to get a sense of which way works best for you. Alternatively, you might deliberately explore whether a particular issue responds better by addressing little bytes or larger chunks of issues.

# NOTES

## Bundling issues

When people are in a supportive situation, such as in ongoing therapy; have experience with and confidence in using WHEE; and/or I feel (through clinical assessment and intuition) that they are emotionally stable, I will often recommend that they work on several related issues at once. I have found this useful myself.

*Example 8:*

> *Recently, I felt inner resistance and doubts about trusting and relying on people to help me. Asking my inner self where this was coming from, I was led immediately to re-examine some of my early childhood issues. I had worked repeatedly through the years on many aspects of my feelings about my parents not being available to me in childhood. Here was yet another layer of these old hurts, asking to be released from the place where it had been locked away by my child mind.*
>
> *As I began to use WHEE (from the perspective of my inner child) on "There is no one here to catch me if I fall," feelings about my mother and father came welling up out of some recess of a closet that I had not fully cleared previously. Rather than working on my feelings towards each of them separately, I chose to bundle them together, because I felt very similarly about both. I left off my focus on "no one here to catch me" at a SUDS of 8; shifted to "Even though my mother and father aren't there for me in ways that I need them to be; and I feel there is no one here today I can ask to help me…" This shifted rapidly from a SUDS of 9 down to zero. Returning to "no one here to catch me," I found it had gone down to a 2, and quickly came down to zero with another round of WHEE.*

Bundling issues may or may not work in any given situation. I recommend it mostly after clients have been using WHEE for a while on individual issues and have a fairly clear sense of how WHEE works for them. Bundling could be confusing if used before this, because it could make it difficult to sort the sources for resistance, due to the variety of issues being addressed. (See also *partializing*, above, the opposite of bundling.)

# NOTES

**Suggestions:**

Again, I encourage you to explore whether addressing single issues or bundled issues feels better to you. This may differ also with the particular issues you are addressing.

Staying flexible and being willing to explore different options at different times with different issues will give you the best range of benefits from WHEE.

# NOTES

## Journaling

***Journal the exact words that you use in your affirmations.*** This can be a help if you find that your SUDS is not changing. It could be that your unconscious is not resonating with the words you have chosen. You can often resume progress by shifting and changing the ways you identify and name your issues and the ways you state the positives you are working to install. Another way the journal can be helpful is if you had a particularly successful rounds of WHEE but were interrupted and want to return to finish the good work you started.

***Journaling helps you to see and follow your progress***. Writing down your experiences, thoughts, feelings, dreams and transpersonal explorations helps to keep your focus. It also provides a diary of your growth and changes.

***Journaling as a diary of your inner experiences is another form of healing.***

> *Those who do not have power over the story that dominates their lives - the power to retell it, rethink it, deconstruct it, joke about it, and change it as times change - truly are powerless, because they cannot think new thoughts.*
>
> – Salman Rushdie

Journaling can be an outlet for feelings and a great aid to sorting out our problems. Writing out one's story and feelings has a cathartic effect, allows a person to consider the problems at a distance, provides perspective as one reviews journaled materials from the past and much more.

Most people find that a hand written journal feels better and gives them a greater sense of personal connection with the materials they are writing about. The advantage of computer journaling is that it allows for easy edits, cross-references, and scanning for particular entries.

## Suggestions:

I cannot encourage you enough to experiment and explore with your journaling to discover what works best for you. And again, be prepared to find that there may be issues or times in your life when journaling suits or doesn't suit your preferences.

# NOTES

## WHEE as a doorway to transpersonal dimensions

*Wholistic healing* addresses body, emotions, mind, relationships (with other people and the environment) and spirit. WHEE helps us to address all of these levels of our being, if we choose to use it in its fullest potential.

*Body* is addressed with WHEE through attending to what symptoms are telling us; through muscle testing; and through treatment of symptoms. Within Wholistic perspectives, body is energy as well as matter. Biological energies can be used to identify issues on all levels of our being that can be helped through various forms of bioenergy healing. This can be done through self-healing and with the help of spiritual healers (Therapeutic Touch, Healing Touch, Reiki, prayers and other forms of healing) and through various forms of complementary/ alternative therapies. (See more on these approaches in Benor, Healing Research, Volumes I and II – details below.)

*Emotions, mind and relationships with other people* are the primary focus of WHEE, discussed above. When viewed with a wholistic perspective, there can be a more healing quality to how we deal with these levels of issues, as discussed below.

*Relationships with the environment* include awarenesses of positive and negative *vibrations* or biological energies that can promote health or contribute to illnesses; a sense of responsibility to protect and restore the environment; and a sense of being an essential part of *Gaia,* the entire planet. (See more on body, emotions, mind and relationships in Benor, Healing Research, Volume 2 – details below.)

*Spirit* informs and inspires every aspect of our lives. Awareness of the transcendent gives us perspectives that extend from before our birth to after our physical death. We may be able to understand the lessons we are learning in this life as part of lessons on many other levels: our own past and future lives; relationships to other people with whom we have shared lessons across many lifetimes; communications with spirits of people who have passed on to existence in other dimensions; transpersonal healings; relationships with all other living beings on our planet and with Gaia, our planet itself; and our relationship with the Infinite Source (call this God, the All, or whatever you find that fits for you).

From these perspectives, problems in our lives take on very different proportions and meanings. Prayer becomes a more meaningful communica-

# NOTES

tion with the All; our issues and challenges can be seen as soul lessons; and our mission in life takes on broader and deeper meanings. (See much more on personal spirituality in Benor, Healing Research, Volume III -details below).

## Suggestions:

In your journaling, pay attention to experiences that speak to you of the transcendent. These may come to your awareness as prayers that are answered; synchronicities, those magical 'coincidences' that tell us there is more meaning to life than we can comprehend; healings that are gifted to you by others; and healings that you are able to offer others.

See more on the inter-relationships between all of the wholistic levels at www.ijhc.org - clicking on any of the icons at the top of the first page.

# NOTES

## Proxy healing with WHEE

*In transpersonal healings it is possible to offer and receive healing across time and space*. For instance, I have had excellent results with 'proxy' (also called 'surrogate') uses of WHEE. In proxy treatments, the person receiving the treatment focuses her or his awareness on another person who is intended to receive the treatment – while that person is not physically present with the person offering the treatment. Therapists may practice the treatment on themselves as proxies for their clients, or may have another person act as a surrogate for the person who is to receive the treatment. (While this may seem far-fetched, it has an excellent basis in research as *distant healing* (Benor 2001).

*Example 9:*

> I visited a healer who was baby-sitting a six-year old boy who has developmental delays and appeared to have mild autism. He was severely frightened by the healer's two dogs, which were lively and playful. He had been in the healer's home several times previously, and was constantly on the alert, if not alarmed, by any approach of the animals to within several feet. Within minutes of proxy tapping for his fears of the animals, he was markedly less fearful, and within a few more minutes he was even able to pet the quieter dog. He had never been that calm before in the animals' presence, and certainly would not have petted them.

*Ethical considerations in proxy healing and other distant healings* are important. Healing is a potent intervention and can bring about changes on all levels of a person's being. Distant healing has been shown to produce measurable effects. (See Benor, *Healing Research*, Volume 1.) Ethical practice requires that we ask permission of anyone to whom we are intending to send healing, or obtain permission from a responsible parent or guardian if they are incapable of giving permission themselves because they are minors or not in a mental state in which to respond. (See fuller discussion of ethics in healing on the www.CouncilForHealing.org site)

## Suggestions:

When a person needing WHEE is unable to be present, and you have permission from them (or from a responsible parent or guardian) to offer your treatment, you can use WHEE as described above. Write down the time

# NOTES

at which you do this. Often, when it is successful, the person receiving the treatment will experience a shift in their symptoms at or around the same time. However, distant treatments may transcend time as well as space, so you might find that the recipient reports a distinct and unexpected shift at a different time from when you were doing the WHEE.

# NOTES

## Developing intuition

*Intuition comes as a certain feeling or a still voice.... If you use your intuition, you will know the very purpose for which you exist in this world; and when you find that, you find happiness.*
                                        – Paramahansa Yogananda

***Intuition*** includes past experience that can be pulled up on the screen of your awareness as *pattern recognition*; *psychic information* from telepathy, clairsentience, pre- and retro-cognition; and *transcendent/ spiritual awarenesses*. Everyone has a measure of intuitive abilities – even skeptics who don't believe in intuition and psychic awarenesses.

WHEE will help you to develop your intuition in a variety of ways:

***Dialoguing with your symptoms*** sharpens your awareness of your inner wisdom. Your unconscious mind knows everything about you. By connecting with this store of inner knowledge, you open doors to access this part of yourself whenever you need it.

***Using the SUDS*** helps you to connect with your inner awareness of the intensity of positive and negative feelings. This heightens your sensitivity to feelings, lessens fears about feelings, and informs your unconscious mind that it no longer has to bury unpleasant feelings or urge you to run away from them. When your unconscious mind isn't putting up lots of walls to 'protect' you from the skeletons in its closets, it is more easily accessible.

***Muscle testing***, which gives you access to your unconscious mind, can help you deliberately access your intuition.

***Dreams*** provide windows into intuitive awarenesses. Dreams are metaphoric expressions of whatever is going on inside you. Interpreting dreams is a challenge and an art. You are the only one who can say what your dreams mean to you, though a wise counselor can suggest possible interpretations that you might not have considered. Similarly, books on dreams can suggest other ways of considering the meanings of your dreams – though they cannot interpret them for you because you are unique and no book can provide the precise meanings that fit your life situation.

Dreams often include transpersonal elements. These may have a special quality to them  that feels  like  it is  coming from outside yourself;  they may

# NOTES

include communications from other people – living and deceased; and they may contain elements of precognition.

**Suggestions:**

By focusing on your intuition, you will encourage it to speak more and you will become more open and aware of when it is wanting to speak to you.

Record when you have spontaneous intuitive feelings that guide you to do or not do particular things that you would otherwise not have considered.

Keep a record of instances where you deliberately ask questions and seek intuitive answers. This will help you improve your focus, your phrasing of questions, and your confidence in using your intuition.

# NOTES

If you wish to recall your dreams, keep a pen and paper or a tape recorder by the bedside. Write down whatever you recall of your dreams, even if it is only a fragment of an image or a feeling, immediately when you waken. If you wait even the few moments it takes to relieve your bladder, you may lose your recall for the dream.

Journaling your dreams is extremely helpful in your personal development.

# NOTES

## Muscle testing to connect with intuition

*Intellect must be balanced by intuition and caring, so that information will be used appropriately, for the good of all and for the future generations.*

– Kenneth Cohen (2003, p. 79)

Muscle testing has been used for more than a century in hypnotherapy. The *ideomotor response* invites the unconscious mind to communicate its knowledge, bypassing the ordinary blocks between conscious and unconscious awarenesses. A hypnotist will suggest that one of a person's fingers will move to indicate *yes* in response to a question, and another finger will move to indicate *no.* This method requires the intervention of a therapist.

More recently, Applied Kinesiology was developed as another therapist-generated treatment, focused on acupuncture meridians. Meridians influence local muscles. If a particular muscle is weak, it indicates that its meridian is weak. Treating this meridian can then correct problems in the body organs that are associated with that meridian. Gradually, aspects of AK have come to be used also for accessing intuition and for self-healing.

Muscle testing is particularly helpful for accessing your intuitive wisdom, using your body as an indicator for yes/ no answers to your questions. Several approaches are in common use.

***The Bi-Digital O-Ring Test (BDORT)*** – Hold the tips of your left thumb and little finger together, forming an 'O' or ring. Hook your right thumb through this ring, just where the left thumb and finger are touching and see how firmly you have to pull in order to break the grip of these fingers. Now, ask yourself, "What does my *yes* feel like?" and repeat the process, noting any change in the strength of your grip. Repeat the process, checking the strength of your grip while you are asking yourself, "What does my *no* feel like?" Most people will find there is a distinct difference in the strength of their grip with a *yes* and a *no*. Most frequently, people find that the *yes* is stronger.

***Index finger muscle testing*** – While sitting, rest your left hand on your leg, near your knee. Raise your index finger. Use your right index finger to press down on your raised left index finger, to check the strength of your left finger. Now, repeat this while you think of a question that can be answered with a *yes* or a *no*. For instance, you might ask, "Is chocolate good for me?" (You may substitute any other food you have cravings for.) See if you notice

# NOTES

any change in the strength of your left index finger. Weakness generally indicates a *no*, strength signifies *yes*.

***Thumbnail muscle testing*** – Gently rub your first finger back and forth across the nail of your thumb, while asking "What is my *yes*?" and "What is my *no*?" Note any differences in what you feel with your finger. Extend this to practice with other questions. You might say out loud, "Today is ___" (stating the correct day) and explore the feeling of your finger running across your thumbnail. Then say, "Today is ___" (stating the wrong day) and again check your sensation. The *yes* usually feels smoother, but this is a very individual modality, with a wider range of variations than many other muscle testing approaches. (This is the method I prefer personally.)

***Your arm as your indicator*** – Extend your arm out to your side, parallel with the floor. Have a friend test the strength of your arm muscles by pressing down on your wrist to establish your baseline strength to resist his pushing down. (She should press firmly, but not so hard as to 'break' your position.) Think silently to yourself of a situation that makes you feel sad. (Don't tell your friend what you are doing, so there will be no question that your arm is being pressed down either more or less firmly according to her expectations.) Note whether your muscle strength is different when she pushes down a second time, as you are focused on sadness. Then rest your arm a moment and have her press down on your wrist again while you're thinking of something that makes you happy. Note the strength of your arm. See the next paragraph for the most common responses to this sort of testing. (Many therapists use arm muscle testing as their way of eliciting ideomotor responses to help you to answer diagnostic and therapeutic questions.)

Sadness usually produces weakness; happiness strengthens the muscles. Occasionally an individual will have a habitually reverse response. A woman I worked with once shared her experience: "I grew up in a tough neighborhood. I taught myself to be tough if I was sad and never to cry, because if I cried they made fun of me." Her arm was much stronger when she was sad.

***Imagery instead of muscle testing*** – Bring up a blank screen in your mind's eye. Ask your unconscious mind to insert an image on the screen that stands for *yes*. After receiving your *yes* image, blank the screen again. Then ask for a *no* image.

***Pendulums and dowsing rods for muscle testing*** – For centuries, people have demonstrated the ability to note the movement of a dowsing rod or

114

NOTES

pendulum to answer questions intuitively. While initially these were used to locate underground water for wells, their use has broadened to answering the same spectrums of questions as in any other form of muscle testing. It is clear that these are muscle testing devices because when a person's hand is rested on the edge of a table, the pendulum will not move to answer *yes* or *no* questions.

## Suggestions:

You can make a pendulum by tying any small object, such as a ring from your finger, onto one end of the thread. Make a loop in the other end and place it around the first joint of your finger. Hold the pendulum out so that it can swing freely. Ask, "what is my 'yes'?" and observe the movement of the pendulum. Note the direction of the swing. For some people this is a linear swing; for others a circular swing. Then ask, "what is my 'no'?" Usually, this will be a swing in the opposite direction to the 'yes.'

You can make a dowsing rod by cutting off a section of a narrow gage metal coat hanger and bending it to an 'L' shape, making certain that the short end of the 'L' is very straight and clear of any bends. Place a piece of a plastic drinking straw over the short end of the 'L' so that it will swivel when you hold it in your hand. Holding a single rod in one hand, tilt it very slightly so that it points directly out in front of you. Ask, "what is my 'yes'?" and observe the movement of the rod. Note the direction of it points to. Then ask, "what is my 'no'?" Usually, this will be a swing in the opposite direction to the 'yes.' You may prefer to do this with a rod in each hand, observing their movements in response to your questions.

Any time you want to use the pendulum or dowsing rod, before you start to ask other questions, check to be certain your 'yes' and 'no' are consistent with previous use of the instrument. If not, then do some grounding exercises before proceeding.

Next, ask, "Is it for my highest good and the highest good of all to be asking this question now?" You should get a 'yes' answer if you are to proceed.

# NOTES

**Muscle testing can be used as a 'truth meter.'** Having established your *yes* and *no* responses concerning neutral issues, you can proceed to ask yourself questions about your physical or psychological wellbeing. Simpler questions might concern whether various foods or medicines are likely to be helpful or harmful. We often find that the foods we particularly crave are the ones that muscle testing will indicate are bad for us. Chocolate, coffee and white sugar are frequent culprits. You may also explore more complicated questions, such as whether or not it is for your highest good to engage in certain experiences or relationships, or whether psychological factors could be contributing to a stress state or illness. Any question at all can be posed, as long as it is simplified to allow a *yes* or *no* reply or series of replies.

Record your questions before or as you ask them. Your unconscious mind and higher self are extremely literal and will respond to the exact words you used in framing your questions. If you feel the answers you are getting are too illogical or feel wrong, ask your question in different ways.

*Example 10:*

> *Frank, a middle-aged participant in one of my workshops, became agitated and tearful when he started using muscle testing. We asked him what was upsetting him. He replied, "I have cancer, and I asked, 'Will I die?' and the answer was yes. I asked several times and the answer was still yes."*
>
> *Several of the other participants in the group started to laugh. Though I was startled by this laughter, I then realized that the answer to Frank's question could only be yes – for anyone who asked that question!*

What Frank really wanted to ask was, "Will I die *soon* from this cancer?"

So be very precise and specific in asking your questions!

I repeat here the cautions discussed in detail in Healing Research, Volume II, Chapter 2: One must be extremely careful in interpreting the results of muscle testing. As with any diagnostic procedure (intuitive or physical), there will always be a percentage of false positive and false negative findings.

# NOTES

***Several ways to reduce the risk of error in muscle testing*** include:

1. *Use common sense and logical reasoning* to analyze information that arises intuitively. Don't act rashly on the basis of intuitive impressions that contradict reason, and reject intuitive urges that go counter to ethics and moral principles.

2. *Examine your introspective, emotional and intuitive responses* to the information provided through muscle testing. The information you bring up may be similar to dream imagery, which can be distorted. That is, the *yes* you receive may be a yes to part of a question rather than to the whole question. When in doubt, consult trusted, wise family, friends and professional therapists.

3. *Record the precise words you use in asking the questions*, so they can be re-evaluated in the light of later analysis. This then allows you to tweak the questions for greater clarity and confidence in the answers.

4. *Reversals* may occur in the muscle testing. Our usual *yes* response may be expressed by our muscles as weakness instead of strength, and our *no* as increased strength. This can happen when we are distressed, ungrounded, in an environment that has dissonant bioenergies, and in other circumstances where we cannot identify the cause. If you sense that this is happening, ground yourself again and do some brain balancing exercises. This will usually stop the reversals.

5. When there are persistent questions and unclarity about results obtained with muscle testing, use multiple readings and supplement them with readings by others, preferably by people such as clinicians who are experienced and expert in the use of these methods.

## Suggestions:

Start out asking simple questions for which you know the answers. Explore which form of muscle testing works best for you.

Initially, you may be more confident in your muscle responses if your work with another person. State out loud, "My name is _____ (correct name)" while you have this person test your arm strength as you extend your arm straight out to your side, horizontally to the floor. Then state

# NOTES

out loud, "My name is _____(incorrect name)" while your arm strength is tested. See what differences you note.

You may have difficulty believing that the person testing your strength isn't pushing harder when s/he knows the incorrect answer. Check this out by either answering the questions silently to yourself or by taking a question to which the answer will not be known by this person, such as the last digit of your social security number.

Play with this at any and every opportunity – it can be fun as well as educational.

Write down the answers you get to your questions. Be careful to note the specific words that you use to ask the questions, because your unconscious mind – the source and filter for many of the answers you will get – is very literal. For instance, "Am I angry because my father beat me as a child?" may get a *yes* muscle testing answer, but may not be as helpful as if you ask, "Is my chronic anger totally due to my father beat me as a child?" There may be other answers, sometimes several factors, that are relevant – which you might overlook if you ask too narrow a question. You may also be unhappy in your job, frustrated in a relationship, or eating foods that make you more irritable.

NOTES

## Transpersonal intuition

Our intuition can reach anywhere and anywhen. Everybody has some measure of intuitive abilities. Even skeptics have been found to demonstrate intuition – though they tend to use it to confirm their disbeliefs. (See Healing Research, Volume I, Chapter 3 for a discussion on telepathy, clairsentience, precognition and retrocognition.)

We can use our intuition to ask questions about our health problems; foods, supplements and treatments that are under consideration; and future events. We can ask questions about other people. Therapists will often use this to access their intuition in order to help clients. In such uses, the ethical considerations mentioned above under *proxy healings* are relevant.

'Blind' readings by a trusted, intuitive person can be particularly reassuring when the answers turn out to be congruent with your understanding of the situation. You can also ask another person to give a *yes* or *no* answer to a question that you are thinking about, without telling that person what the question is. This eliminates biases of familiarity with a situation, expectations, anxieties or fears. However, as with any intuitive exploration, we must always be cautious because intuition is an art as much as a science. There is always a percent of correct and incorrect answers.

The help of a knowledgeable clinician can be invaluable. Clinicians trained in muscle testing know the ways in which innate characteristics and learned patterns of beliefs and behaviors tend to cluster and manifest – both physically and psychologically. Clinicians may identify psychological issues that we ourselves are blind to – particularly around traumatic experiences that we have buried in our unconscious mind, and relating to habit patterns that we are blind to. Good psychotherapists will know ways to help unravel the complex structures of defenses built up over a lifetime of human interactions, and bioenergy therapists may recognize blocks or over-activities in various meridians that would not be apparent or even suspected by anyone who is unfamiliar with these patterns.

*Where there is doubt or question you must proceed with the greatest caution when using these techniques.* Your unconscious expectations, hopes, wishes and fears may all influence your self-explorations – leading you to ask questions in ways that provide answers more comfortable to your wishes and expectations, or conversely, to avoid questions that might produce uncomfortable answers. The same may apply for therapists, whose own unresolved issues may make them blind, insensitive or uncomfortable with particular client problems.

# NOTES

**Suggestions:**

Play with this at every opportunity. I repeat myself here because this is really important. Write down the answers you get to your questions. Be careful to note the specific words that you use to ask the questions, because your unconscious mind – the source and filter for many of the answers you will get – is very literal. For instance, "Am I going to meet my true love?" may get a *yes* answer, but you may be thinking, "Am I going to meet this person tomorrow night at the dance?" and your unconscious mind may be answering from the perspective of your whole life ahead of you... unless you ask the question with "tomorrow night at the dance" as a part of your statement of the question.

You might ask, "Is this cantaloupe ripe and juicy and sweet?" or "Is it better for me to be in the right lane or the left lane as I'm approaching this light?" Questions like these will give you the immediate feedback so that you learn to understand and trust your intuition. Remember, though, that you must always be specific with your questions. "Is it better to be in the right or left lane" can be interpreted in various ways. You might be focused on getting somewhere as quickly as possible. Your unconscious mind might be focused on getting you through the traffic light safely, avoiding a car that is going to come barreling through the intersection, so that not moving as quickly may be better.

The perspective from which you ask the question may give you different answers. Again, the wording you use is important. "Should I buy this _____ [car, house, pineapple]?" is a very vague way to ask the question, because "should" can have many shades of meanings and interpretations. "Will I be happy with my purchase of this _____?" or "Will this _____ last for __ years of use and give me good service and satisfaction?" might be the ways you could get more clear and useful answers.

"Will it be for my highest good to buy this _____?" invites a transpersonal context for your Q/A. "

The regular inclusion of the transpersonal sets your questions and your life on more spiritual pathways, framing of your question in a phrasing such as: "Will it be for my highest good *and the highest good of all* to _____?"

# NOTES

## A spectrum of problems helped by WHEE

WHEE has been hugely successful for several reasons:

- WHEE takes a fraction of the time that EFT and other MBTs require.

- WHEE allows for much greater flexibility in working on target problems within a session because it is so rapid. If a child is successful but the parent is not, or vice versa, there is plenty of time to explore alternative symptoms or alternative methods of addressing these.

- WHEE is gentle and does not cause intense emotional releases, although it does thoroughly and permanently clear the emotions associated with old hurts.

- WHEE is better accepted and the compliance outside the therapy room is much higher because of this simplicity.

- WHEE works marvelously well and rapidly on problems that may have been present for a long time and may not have responded to other therapies, such as pains, cravings and allergies, though it may take several days to be effective for the latter.

- WHEE is tremendously empowering, as it is so simple and so rapidly effective in self-healing.

I find that 85-90 percent of clients obtain immediate benefits from WHEE. When they practice this for their problems at home, there is almost universal success. Below is a spectrum of problems that have responded well to WHEE.

Underline or note on the opposite page any of these items that are relevant to you.

- *Fears* – Anxieties about new activities or new places, including visits to dentists and doctors; fears of flying; fears of insects, snakes, pets and larger animals, heights; test anxieties; performance anxieties, such as speaking in class or in public; specific fears following frightening or traumatic experiences; anxieties and fears about recurring experiences such as medical treatments, shifting between homes of parents who are not living together (See article on 'Re-entry problems' referenced at the end of this manual); calming after waking from a nightmare; dealing with underlying anxieties and post traumatic residues associated with nightmares.

# NOTES

- **Phobias, including school avoidance** – even in severe cases where the child previously had to be dragged from the car by his parents and held by the vice principal so he wouldn't run back to the car. Milder fears, such as those marked by procrastination, respond well too.

- **Post-traumatic Stress Disorders (PTSD)** – are very responsive to WHEE, which can help with residual traumatic memories, panic attacks, nightmares, temper outbursts and more.

- **Angers** – Preventive use of WHEE is best, emptying the 'bucket of old angers' so that it doesn't overflow when new angers are stuffed inside. Once people have practiced using WHEE when they are not angry, then they can use WHEE at times of upsets, such as releasing anger and calming while sitting in a time out chair; addressing fears and hurts that may be associated with the angers.

- **Insomnia** – responds wonderfully well, even when it has been present for a long time.

- **Motion sickness and morning sickness of pregnancy** – can respond immediately and can be eliminated.

- **Emotional pains** – Emotional distress after painful emotional experiences – both recent and from distant past, such as parental conflicts, separation or divorce; worries over family stresses such as illness, injuries and financial issues; bereavement.

- **Physical pains of all sorts** – These have responded rapidly to WHEE, including tension headaches, migraines, stomach aches, pains after injuries, arthritis. CAUTION: Pain may be a signal from the body that people are 'up tight' over a stressful situation and are in distress, but may be unaware of what it is that is stressing them. It is important to consider such possibilities carefully before working on removing the pain.

- **Cravings** – For sweets, food, drugs, thrills, have all responded to WHEE.

- **Allergies** – to animals, pollens and other allergens; asthma. Allergies may respond within minutes or may take several weeks of regular WHEE use to dissipate.

# NOTES

*Example 11:*

- *Tony visited a home where I was also present. As he came in the door, he immediately apologized that he was likely to have to leave early because he had forgotten to bring along his medicine to protect him from sneezing and coughing because of his cat allergy. He was open to learning WHEE and with just a ten minute session found that he was symptom-free for the full three hour visit.*

- ***Weight loss*** - for reducing, eliminating, transforming:
  Food cravings – for specific foods and in general
  Stress responses – allowing systematic transformation of negative responses that
    often initiate comfort eating
  Residues of old traumas – from mild discomfort at awkward memories to major
    post-traumatic stress disorder (PTSD)
  Issues around self-image and self-esteem
  Meta-issues of habits around being overweight and how to be in the world – heavy
    or not heavy; lighter or not lighter

- ***Reducing side effects and the need for medications*** – both in the reduction in severity of the issues for which the medications are prescribed (anxiety, pain, allergies, insomnia, etc.), and in harmonizing the response to medications, such as chemotherapy, reducing side effects for which other medications are prescribed.

- ***Relationships, social issues, performance anxieties, low self-confidence*** – common issues of teens – respond dramatically well to WHEE. This is an extension of the uses of WHEE into beliefs and disbeliefs about our abilities to deal with issues.

- ***Family members' anxieties and distress*** – There have been excellent responses in anxieties raised by children's, partners' and parents' issues; anxieties not caused by the children but impacting the children because children pick up on parents' worries or because parents have a shorter fuse; anxieties and stresses of relatives dealing with a family member's chronic illness.

I used to worry that if people released their symptoms and illnesses by using a rapidly effective technique such as WHEE, they would develop other symptoms because of underlying problems that were causing the symptoms.

NOTES

This has not been the case. It appears that WHEE releases whatever is ready to be released, below the surface as well as on the surface. As I work with more and more people with WHEE, I am more and more convinced that the symptoms are the tips of the icebergs of issues that are asking for attention and release. The symptoms are not separate from the issues, they are a very much parts of them. Often the symptoms are metaphors for the issues, as when a pain in the neck is begging us to look at who in our lives is a pain in the neck for us; a urinary problem might be saying we are 'pissed off' at someone; and a cardiac problem could be speaking of an emotional heartache. By addressing the body metaphor, the underlying issue is also addressed. (See much more on this in Benor, Healing Research, Volume II – details below.)

> *Mostly, people change not because they see the light*
> *but because they feel the heat.*
> — David Grudermeyer

**Suggestions:**

Write down things that bother, worry or frighten you about any of the above issues.

# NOTES

Having written down your spontaneous responses to these questions, here are some structured questions to guide you further in your explorations of issues for which WHEE may be helpful to you.

## Anxieties, Fears and Phobias

Do you have:

Anxieties or fears about new activities or new places ____
List specific places and things about these places that have bothered you.

Fears of flying or of other travel ____
List specific times and factors about travel that have been unpleasant or uncomfortable.

Anxieties about being on time or being late ____
What places or events have been trying experiences for you? Are there regular times in your schedule that you worry about this?

Visits to dentists or doctors ____
List specific experiences you have had that have been unpleasant, painful, frightening, or traumatic.

Fears of insects, snakes, pets and larger animals ____
Write down fears you have and things that have happened to you which started these fears. For instance, were you ever stung by a bee? Bitten by a dog?

Fears of heights ____
e.g. Ladders; stairways; looking out a window of a tall building; bridges; flying

# NOTES

Fears of cramped or narrow spaces ____

e.g. Elevators; seats that are not on the aisle; small or crowded rooms; having the door to a room closed


Fears of how people will accept you ____

e.g. Speaking in public; interviews; approaching members of the opposite sex; salespeople

Test anxieties ____ e.g. Do you freeze when faced by an exam? Perform poorly on exams even though you have studied and know the materials?


Performance anxieties ____

e.g. Do you worry how you will succeed in sports, presentations, study, work or volunteer projects?


Fears following frightening or traumatic experiences? ____


Post-traumatic stress disorder ____

PTSD can include fears of things that are similar to those in which you experienced the trauma; sensitivity and stress with loud noises; panic attacks; excessive anger with minor provocations; temper outbursts; difficulty falling asleep or staying asleep; nightmares; night sweats; flashbacks


Children who have difficulties handling shifts between homes of parents who are not living together ____


Children who are afraid of going to school ____

This can be expressed as avoidance of doing the work for a specific class or teacher; procrastinating leaving home in the morning; avoiding or refusing to go to school, using any and every excuse; refusing to enter the school building or classroom

NOTES

## Angers

Do you have frequent, excessive irritability, anger or temper outbursts with minimal provocations ____

This could be with specific people such as a family member, partner, employer; employee; or it could be with specific types of people, such as authority figures, any member of the opposite sex, or people with particular characteristics (appearance, mannerisms, accents)

Do you hold angers inside and simmer over them____

## Insomnia

Do you have difficulty

Falling asleep on going to bed or after waking during the night ____

Staying asleep ____

Being bothered by nightmares ____

Waking too early in the morning ____

## Motion sickness and morning sickness of pregnancy

Do you have severe queasiness ____ nausea ____ vomiting ____

Do you have these symptoms even when you remember being in a vehicle or being pregnant____

140

# NOTES

_____

_____

_____

_____

_____

_____

_____

_____

_____

_____

_____

_____

_____

_____

### *Emotional pains*

Do you have:

Worries or distress over current stresses ____
e.g. personal or family member illness or injuries; conflicts with a partner or family member; financial issues; bereavement

Emotional distress from painful emotional experiences in the distant past ____
e.g. when you remember your parents or other family members arguing or fighting; separating; divorcing; remarrying; being ill or injured; moving from one home to another;

### *Physical pains*

Do you suffer from:

Pains of recent origins
    Muscle strains, injuries or surgery ____

Chronic pains ____
    Muscle pains such as: tension headaches, backaches ____
    Pains persisting long after injuries or surgery ____
    Arthritis, migraines, irritable bowel syndrome ____

### *Allergies*

Are you allergic to
    Specific animals ____ List these:
    Pollens ____
    Other allergens ____

Do you have
    Asthma ____
    Eczema ____

# NOTES

*Cravings*

Do you have a problem resisting
Sweets \_\_\_\_
Food \_\_\_\_
Smoking \_\_\_\_
Marijuana \_\_\_\_
Alcohol \_\_\_\_
Cocaine \_\_\_\_
Other drugs \_\_\_\_
Sex (in inappropriate contexts) \_\_\_\_
Stimulation that is excessive
Taking unusual risks with your body \_\_\_\_
Provoking, teasing or angering people \_\_\_\_
Using video or hand-held games \_\_\_\_
Watching TV when it is just chewing gum for the mind \_\_\_\_

*Reducing side effects and the need for medications*

Are you taking medications for symptoms or problems for which WHEE might be helpful, so that if these problems are bothering you less, you may need less medications or no medications at all? e.g.
Anxiety, stress or panic disorders \_\_\_\_
Depression, dysthymia (lack of joy, bordering on depression) \_\_\_\_
Chronic pains, arthritis, irritable bowel syndrome \_\_\_\_
Reactive hypertension, with blood pressure rising due anxiety or stress \_\_\_\_
Insomnia \_\_\_\_
Allergies \_\_\_\_

Are you taking medications or receiving treatments that produce uncomfortable side effects, which WHEE can reduce or eliminate?
Hormone replacement therapy \_\_\_\_
Antihypertensive medications \_\_\_\_
Antidepressants, mood stabilizers \_\_\_\_
Chemotherapy \_\_\_\_
Radiotherapy \_\_\_\_

# NOTES

### *Weight loss*

Have you had difficulties with
   Food cravings – for specific foods and in general ____
   Stress responses or habits that initiate frequent comfort eating ____
   Reducing diets ____
   Issues around self-image and self-esteem ____
   Issues around being accepted or rejected by others ____

### *Relationships, social issues*

Are you anxious, depressed or angry over your relationships
   With parents, brothers or sisters, children or partners
   With teachers, students or fellow students ____
   With your boss, fellow workers, employees ____
   With clients ____

Are you upset over
   Not achieving the recognition you feel you deserve ____
   Not being able to say "No" to unreasonable expectations or
   demands ____

### *Low self-confidence*

Do you hesitate to
   Express your views and opinions at home ____
   Express your views and opinions at work ____
   Assert your authority at home ____
   Assert your authority at work ____
   Say what you are thinking or feeling if you think others may
   disagree with you ____
   Wear clothes that you prefer because you are anxious about
   criticisms ____
   Ask for help ____
   Ask for attention and caring ____
   Say 'No' if you feel you are not up to meeting someone's request or
   expectations____

# NOTES

## Dealing with blocks in using WHEE

Where WHEE doesn't work, the most frequent problem are:

1. We have not targeted the problem accurately in the affirmation.

2. We have forgotten to massage the releasing point when there is a block in the process.

3. We have meta-anxiety or other meta-problems that are blocking us from releasing.

4. We may note that the memories of traumas are not fading as we work with WHEE. This is an incorrect expectation, as it is the negative feelings *about* the memory that fade, not the necessarily our factual memory of events.

If the above do not apply, the few remaining clients may respond to the EFT routine or other MBT approaches.


## Suggestions:

Write down the blocks you encounter and how you resolve them. This item in your journaling may be helpful to you in future instances of blocks, providing clues to where the blocks are and how to clear them.

Find other people who are using WHEE and ask them what they might do with the issue that is not shifting. Often, a fresh perspective will offer clues to new approaches that will get you around the blocks.

Participate in Dr. Benor's telephone seminars for people who use WHEE for themselves or for their clients/ respants/ patients

Dr. Benor is available for consultation by phone or email, per the contact details at the front and back of this workbook.

# NOTES

## Additional benefits with using WHEE

*Most people are about as happy as they make up their minds to be.*
– Ralph Waldo Emerson

**WHEE helps to forgive** others for their transgressions, helps you to forgive yourself for not having done better than your best – at the times when you stuffed feelings into your inner 'bucket,' and to accept that you did the best you could at those times and now are more competent to deal with the residues of the situations that left you with bad feelings.

## Suggestions:

List people who have upset you, about whom you have felt bad and carried resentments.

Ask yourself whether you would like to let go of some of your resentments towards any of these people. If so, put check marks after their names, above.

If you are ready to release these resentments, use WHEE to do this, naming the feelings that arise when you think about them.

Be certain that when you reduce the resentments to zero, you install positives to replace the negatives that you have released.

# NOTES

**WHEE is empowering**. It gives you a clear way to deal with almost any problem you might encounter that raises negative feelings. It helps to clear the 'bucket' of emotional dross – that place inside where you stuff unresolved feelings when you don't know how to resolve a stressful situation.

**Suggestions:**

List your successes in using WHEE here or on a special page in your journal.

Plan a time in your diary to review your successes and add to the list. (Many people find that about once a month is a comfortable interval)

# NOTES

***WHEE develops a sweetening spiral – a positive, self-reinforcing, feedback system*** that encourages and supports further insights, releases of negativity, growth and change. This is the opposite of a vicious circle – where a negative experience generates a negative attitude, which leads to negative behaviors, which beget more negative experiences. (Isn't it odd that there is no common term in our language for the opposite of a vicious circle?)

As you practice self-healing with WHEE, you gain confidence in your abilities to deal with your problems. This enables you to be less afraid of your issues and to deal with them more competently. With an initial success in dealing with your inner stress or old hurts ▯ you feel better ▯ you are less anxious ▯ you have less fear of dealing with old hurts ▯ you take more steps to deal with the hurts ▯ you have more successes ▯ you feel better ▯ etc. Similar sweetening spirals can develop in your social interactions as you progress through the healing process.

Write down

A **positive change in your feelings and beliefs about yourself** that has come from your use of WHEE in various situations (List separate examples in A; B; etc):

A.

B.

C.

D.

Ways in which you have **felt better about yourself** as a result of having changed these feelings and beliefs:

A1.

B1.

C1.

D1

Positive ways in which you have **changed your attitudes and behaviors** as a result of feeling better about yourself:

A2.

B2.

C2.

D2.

# NOTES

**Further positive changes in the ways you feel and believe about yourself** – as a result of your successful changes in attitudes and behaviors:

A3.

B3.

C3.

D3.

Write down:

**Positive changes in your feelings and beliefs** that have come from your use of WHEE:

A.

B.

C.

D.

**Positive ways in which you have changed your attitudes and behaviors towards others** as a result of each of these changes in your feelings and beliefs:

A1.

B1.

C1.

D1

**Positive ways in which others have responded to you** as a result of each of your changes in attitudes and behaviors:

A2.

B2.

C2.

D2.

**Further positive ways in which you have responded towards others**, in response to the changes in ways that others have responded to you:

A3.

B3.

C3.

D3.

# NOTES

***The strong positives that are used at the end of the affirmations*** can create a positive shift in our perspectives and attitudes on life, in and of themselves. Repeating "I love myself wholly and completely" and "God loves and accepts me, wholly and completely and unconditionally" while tapping will strengthen these positive beliefs and awarenesses.

**Suggestions:**

List the positive affirmations you have found helpful:

    e.g. "I love and accept myself wholly and completely"

List the changes you notice in yourself as a result of using these positive affirmations

# NOTES

***Transpersonal awareness is facilitated*** by affirmations that include the Infinite Source and other transpersonal positives.

## Suggestions:

Note ways in which you become more aware that you are a part of a spiritual 'something' that is greater than yourself. In many ways this is not something we learn, so much as something we come to remember through connecting with our intuition, our unconscious mind and our higher self.

# NOTES

**WHEE shifts your attitudes towards problems** so that you can address them as invitations to growth and transformation rather than as worries. Each distressing problem is transformed into a doorway into understanding and clearing the childhood programs that lead you into meta-worries and sap your energies away from addressing the actual concerns.

## Suggestions:

After using WHEE for several weeks, make it a point periodically to write down the shifts you notice in the ways in which you address problems.

Note when and how

You have been able to address specific problems as concerns rather than as worries

You are less upset with yourself over emotions that arise in response to situations that bother you

You are able to identify issues from your past that have contributed to your responses in the present

You have been able to clear the residual feelings from these old feelings, as well as from the situations in the present that have reminded you of them.

162

# NOTES

*WHEE can be a preventive to future problems.*

**Suggestions:**

After using WHEE for several weeks, note the more healing ways in which you now are able to respond to new situations, compared with how you used to respond to them.

164

NOTES

## Theoretical considerations and conclusions

People ask, "How can WHEE work so well and so quickly?" The true answer is that we don't know yet. The best answer I've been able to suggest follows the understanding I have of the ways in which the right and left brain handle traumatic experiences, discussed above (under *Basic Healing Principles*.)

When we do the following, we release our buried hurts:

1. ***Holding the hurts fully within our conscious awareness allows the hurts to dissipate***. This requires that we override our childhood programming to bury what hurts, pretending it is not there, and running away from the buried hurts and from anything in our current life that might remind us of them.

The Sedona method teaches this principle, requiring only the decision to release whatever the problem is and giving ourselves permission to do so.

2. ***Pairing a positive feeling and cognitive awareness with the hurt***. When we hold the positive along with the hurt simultaneously in our awareness, the positive cancels the negative feelings associated with the hurt.

Neurolinguistic Programming (NLP) does this with 'anchors.' A positive and a negative feeling are anchored in the body, and the positive one will cancel out the negative one. The same thing can be done through exercises of mental imagery.

3. ***Activating right and left brain hemispheres*** *while doing (1) and (2) markedly enhances the effects*. It appears as though we can bring the skeletons of old traumas out of the closets in the right brain, while connecting it to the left brain – through the alternating left and right sensory stimulation. As the two hemispheres reconnect in the conscious presence of the traumas, the buried hurts dissipate.

4. ***Involving the body memories and body-mind processes related to difficult issues*** helps enormously in dealing with them. Memories are stored in the body as well as in the brain and spirit. Connecting with the body during therapy will markedly enhance the therapy.

WHEE does all of these and is therefore the most potent self-healing technique I know.

# NOTES

EMDR has a solid basis in research, demonstrating its efficacy in treating stress related disorders. (See details at the end of this Workbook). The MBTs are still in preliminary stages of organizing research. WHEE, drawing from EMDR (though clearly not following the standard EMDR protocols), can claim to have a research base to support its efficacy.

Having advocated for the abbreviated procedure of WHEE, let me step back and add that I do not see this as a 'cure-all.' I find that the MBTs are outstanding for addressing the same spectrum of traumas, fears, pains, allergies, and beliefs that WHEE addresses. The advantage of WHEE is that it is more easily learned, quicker, and has better compliance rates – especially with children.

Some are content to clear their symptoms. Others seek deeper levels of work, which may require more elaborate approaches. I have found Clinton's Matrix Therapy (chakra based) enormously helpful to me personally and to selected clients who want or need deeper levels of work, particularly when there is an openness to including spiritual dimensions in the focus of therapy. I also integrate spiritual awareness and healing, along with many other approaches in my practice, matching the therapy to the individual needs of the client.

# NOTES

## Broader extensions of our individual work

*One cannot really ever overcome the enemy until one has rid oneself of that which is found despicable in the other.*
                                                                        – Stephen Levine

Clearing our own issues 'empties the buckets' of our old hurts and angers. Being free of old emotional residues leaves us less likely to respond with upset, hurt or anger to the behaviors of others. This is helpful in our personal relationships with other people; essential in a therapist-client relationship.

This can also contribute to turning the fires down under the caldrons of sectarian and national angers that lead to broader conflicts. When the collective angers of a nation or society are lessened, we can respond with empathy and understanding in conflict situations, seeking to help the 'others' explore their grievances – with the goal of reaching the best compromises possible.

## PRACTICAL CONSIDERATIONS

The Meridian Based Therapies (WHEE, EFT, TFT and many others in this group) have very limited research to support their efficacy. EMDR has considerable, impressive research showing it is effective in helping adults and children deal with PTSD. By using WHEE, we tap into the EMDR research database. (See selected samples below).

### Status of EMDR acceptance for PTSD

**American Psychiatric Association.** *Practice Guideline for the Treatment of Patients with*

*EMDR has been given the same status as Cognitive Behavioral Therapy (CBT) as an effective treatment of ameliorating symptoms of both acute and chronic PTSD.*

Reference: *Acute Stress Disorder and Posttraumatic Stress Disorder.* Arlington, VA: American Psychiatric Association Practice Guidelines 2004.

## SUGGESTED READING

Benor, Daniel J. WHEE introductory article
www.wholistichealingresearch.com/Articles/Selfheal.asp

Benor, Daniel J. WHEE for trauma and re-entry problems   www.heal911.com/C-6a.asp

Benor, Daniel J. WHEE for children of all ages
www.wholistichealingresearch.com/Articles/WHEE-Child.asp

Benor, Daniel J. The inter-relationships of spirit, relationships (with people and the environment, mind, emotions and body http://wholistichealingresearch.com/srmeb.htm

Cohen, Kenneth S. *Honoring the Medicine: Native American Healing*, New York: Ballantine 2003.

Dennison, PE/ Dennison, G. *Brain Gym Handbook*, Ventura, CA: Educational Kinesiology Foundation 1989.

Dennison, P/ Dennison, GE. *Brain Gym: Teachers Edition, Revised*, Ventura, CA: Edu-Kinesthetics 1994.

Gordon, Thomas. *P.E.T. – Parent Effectiveness Training*, NY: Penguin 1975.
*Excellent on communications between parents; between parents & children.*

Hay, Louise L. *You Can Heal Your Life*, Santa Monica, CA: Hay House 1984.
(*Has list of symptoms' meanings and affirmations to counter them.*)

Laing, Ronald D. *Knots*, NY: Penguin 1970. (See also: *The Divided Self – More technical – Discussions on how we split ourselves off into bits and pieces*)

Siegel, Bernie S. *Love, Medicine & Miracles: Lessons Learned About Self-Healing from a Surgeon's Experience with Exceptional Patients*, New York: Harper & Row 1986.

Stewart, Ian/ Joines, Vann. *TA Today*, Chapel Hill, NC: Lifespace 1991.
(*Excellent, thorough introduction to Transactional Analysis.*)

Siegel, Bernie. *Love, Medicine and Miracles*: Lessons *Learned about Self-Healing from a Surgeon's Experience with Exceptional Patients* NY: Harper & Row 1986.
(*A classic on transformation through illness as an awakening to personal growth.*)

See also list of books, tapes and other Meridian Based Therapy references
www.wholistichealingresearch.com/References/MBTs.htm

## EMDR

Shapiro, Francine. *Eye Movement Desensitization and Reprocessing*, New York: Guildford 1995.

www.emdr.com

### EMDR for Children

Greenwald, Ricky. Eye movement desensitization and reprocessing (EMDR): New hope for children suffering from trauma and loss, www.childtrauma.com/emdrch.html

**Emotional Freedom Technique (EFT)** of Gary Craig www.emofree.com

**Sedona Method** www.Sedona.com

**RESEARCH REFERENCES** - *EMDR*

Acierno, R., Hersen, M., Van Hasselt, et al. Review of the validation and dissemination of eye-movement desensitization and reprocessing: A scientific and ethical dilemma. *Clinical Psychology Review* 1994, *14,* 287-299. ( 'Cautionary' article about EMDR)

Carlson, J. G., Chemtob, C. M., Rusnak, et al. Eye movement desensitization and reprocessing for combat-related post-traumatic stress disorder. *Journal of Traumatic Stress* (in press 1997). .

Chemtob, C. & Nakashima, J. *Eye movement desensitization and rereprocessing (EMDR) treatment for children with treatment resistant disaster related distress.* Presented at the annual meeting of the International Society for Traumatic Stress Studies, San Francisco (1996, November).

Edmond, T. & Rubin, A. *Evaluating the effectiveness of EMDR in reducing trauma symptoms in adult survivors of childhood sexual abuse.* Presented at the annual conference of the EMDR International Association, Denver (1996, June).

Goldstein, A. & Feske, U. Eye movement desensitization and reprocessing for panic disorder: A case series. *Journal of Anxiety Disorders* 1994, *8,* 351-362.

Grainger, R. D., Levin, C., Allen-Byrd, L., et al. An empirical evaluation of eye movement desensitization and reprocessing (EMDR) with survivors of a natural catastrophe. *Journal of traumatic Stress* (in press 1997). .

Greenwald, R. *Using EMDR with children.* Available from EMDR, P.O. Box 51010, Pacific Grove, CA 93950-6010 with formal training 1993.

Greenwald, R. The information gap in the EMDR controversy. *Professional Psychology: Research and Practice* 1996, *27,* 67-72.

Lipke, H. J. *Survey of practitioners trained in eye movement desensitization and reprocessing.* Paper presented at the annual convention of the American Psychological Association, Los Angeles, CA 1994, August.

Marcus, S., Marquis, P., & Sakai, C. *Eye movement desensitization and reprocessing: A clinical outcome study for post-traumatic stress disorder.* Paper presented at the American Psychological Association annual convention, Toronto 1996, August.

Paulsen, S. Eye movement desensitization and reprocessing: Its cautious use in the dissociative disorders. *Dissociation* 1995, *8,* 32-44.

Sanderson, A. & Carpenter, R. (1992). Eye movement desensitization versus image confrontation: A single-session crossover study of 58 phobic subjects. *Journal of Behavior Therapy and Experimental Psychiatry, 23,* 269-275.

Scheck, M. M., Schaeffer, J. A., & Gilette, C. S. (in press). Brief psychological intervention with traumatized young women: The efficacy of eye movement desensitization and reprocessing. *Journal of Traumatic Stress* 1998, 11(1), 25-44.

Shapiro, F. Efficacy of the eye movement desensitization procedure in the treatment of traumatic memories. *Journal of Traumatic Stress* 1989a, *2,* 199-223.

Shapiro, F. Eye movement desensitization: A new treatment for post-traumatic stress disorder. *Journal of Behavior Therapy and Experimental Psychiatry* 1989b, *20,* 211-217.

Shapiro, F. Eye movement desensitization and reprocessing procedure: From EMD to EMD/R - A new treatment model for anxiety and related traumata. *The Behavior Therapist* 1991a, *14,* 133-135.

Shapiro, F. Eye movement desensitization and reprocessing: A cautionary note. *The Behavior Therapist* 1991b, *14,* 188.

Shapiro, F. Eye movement desensitization and reprocessing (EMDR) in 1992. *Journal of Traumatic Stress* 1993a, *6,* 417-421.

Shapiro, F. Eye movement desensitization and reprocessing: A new treatment for anxiety and related trauma. In Lee Hyer (ed.) *Trauma victim: Theoretical and practical suggestions.* Muncie, IN: Accelerated Development 1994.

Shapiro, F. *Eye movement desensitization and reprocessing: Basic principles, protocols and procedures.* New York: Guilford Press 1995.

Shapiro, F. Eye movement desensitization and reprocessing (EMDR): Evaluation of controlled PTSD research. *Journal of Behavior Therapy and Experimental Psychiatry* 1996, *27,* 209-218.

Shapiro, F., Vogelmann-Sine, S., Sine, L. Eye movement desensitization and reprocessing: Treating trauma and substance abuse. *Journal of Psychoactive Drugs* 1994, *26,* 379-391.

Silver, S. M., Brooks, A., Obenchain, J. Treatment of Vietnam war veterans with PTSD: A comparison of eye movement desensitization and reprocessing, biofeedback, and relaxation training. *Journal of Traumatic Stress* 1995, *8,* 337-342.

Sweet, A. A theoretical perspective on the clinical use of EMDR. *The Behavior Therapist* 1995, *18,* 5-6.

Wilson, D. L., Covi, W. G., Foster, S. Eye movement desensitization and reprocessing: Effectiveness and ANS correlates. *Journal of Behavior Therapy and Experimental Psychiatry* 1996, *27,* ?

Wilson, S. A., Becker, L. A., & Tinker, R. H. Eye movement desensitization and reprocessing (EMDR) treatment for psychologically traumatized individuals. *Journal of Consulting and Clinical Psychology* 1995, *63,* 928-937.

(More EMDR research at http://www.emdr.com/efficacy.htm)

## RELATED REFERENCES BY DANIEL BENOR

Benor, Daniel J. *Healing Research: Volume I, Spiritual Healing: Scientific Validation of a Healing Revolution*, Southfield, MI: Vision Publications, 2001.
(*Healers describe their work, research in parapsychology as a context for understanding healing, brief summaries of randomized controlled studies, pilot studies.*)

Benor, Daniel J. *Healing Research: Volume I, Professional Supplement*, Southfield, MI: Vision Publications, 2001.
(*Only the studies -- described in much greater detail, including statistical information.*)

Benor, Daniel J. *Healing Research, Volume II (Professional edition): Consciousness, Bioenergy and Healing*, Medford, NJ: Wholistic Healing Publications, 2004.
(*Self-healing, wholistic complementary/ alternative medicine and integrative care, biological energies, and environmental interactions with bioenergies. Consciousness, Bioenergy and Healing was acknowledged as 'BOOK OF THE YEAR' by the Scientific and Medical Network, UK* )

Benor, Daniel J. *Healing Research, Volume II (Popular edition): How Can I Heal What Hurts?*, Medford, NJ: Wholistic Healing Publications, 2005.
(*Written for the layperson - Same content as Professional edition, plus extra chapter on Self-Healing approaches.*

Benor, Daniel J. *Healing Research, Volume III – Personal Spirituality: Science, Spirit and the Eternal Soul*, Medford, NJ: Wholistic Healing Publications (in press, late 2006).
(*Research on NDE, OBE, spirit survival, reincarnation, spiritual awareness.*)

Benor, Daniel J. *Healing Research, Volume IV - A Synthesis of Recent Research*, Medford, NJ: Wholistic Healing Publications (in press). (*Topical summaries of volumes I-III, with discussion of theories, early synthesis of explanations for healing, in press.*)

Benor, Daniel J. Spiritual healing for mental health, In: Shannon, Scott (ed). *Handbook of Complementary and Alternative Therapies in Mental Health*, San Diego, CA: Academic/Harcourt 2001, 258-267.

http://www.WholisticHealingResearch.com/Articles/MentalHlth-SpirHeal.htm

Benor, Daniel J. Spiritual healing for infertility, pregnancy, labor and delivery, *Complementary Therapies in Nursing and Midwifery* 1996, 2, 106-109.

Benor, Daniel J. Psychotherapy & spiritual healing, *Human Potential,* 1996 (summer), 13-16.

Benor, Daniel J. Further comments on 'loading' and 'telesomatic reactions', *Advances* 1996, 12(2), 71-75.

Benor, Daniel J. Spiritual Healing: A unifying influence in complementary therapies, *Complementary Therapies in Medicine*, 1995, 3(4), 234-238.

Benor, Daniel J. Spiritual healing and psychotherapy, *The Therapist* 1994, 1(4), 37-39 http://www.wholistichealingresearch.com/Articles/SpirHealPT.asp

Benor, Daniel J. Intuitive diagnosis, *Subtle Energies* 1992, 3(2), 41-64 http://www.wholistichealingresearch.com/Articles/IntuitDx.asp.

Benor, Daniel J. A psychiatrist examines fears of healing, *J. Society for Psychical Research* 1990, 56, 287-299 http://www.wholistichealingresearch.com/Articles/FearsHealingPsi.asp.

Benor, Daniel J. Fields and energies related to healing: A review of Soviet & western studies, *Psi Research* 1984, 3(1), 8-15.

Benor, Daniel J. The overlap of psychic 'readings' with psychotherapy, *Psi Research* 1986, 5(1,2), 56-78.

**Daniel J. Benor, MD, ABHM**, has been searching over four decades for ever more ways to peel the onion of life's resistances, to reach the knowing (with the inner knowing of truth which has the feel of rightness) that we are all cells in the body of the Infinite Source.

While his unique area of expertise is spiritual awareness and healing, his principal work is through wholistic healing – addressing spirit, relationships, mind, emotions and body. He is using WHEE, a potent self-healing method, with children and parents (many foster parents) who are dealing with PTSD and other forms of stress, psychological and physical pain, low self-esteem, cravings and other issues.

Dr. Benor founded The Doctor-Healer Network in England and in North America. He is the author of Healing Research, Volumes I-IV and many articles on wholistic, spiritual healing. He is the editor and publisher of the International Journal of Healing and Caring - On Line (www.ijhc.org) and moderator of www.WholisticHealingResearch.com, a major informational website on spiritual awareness, healing and CAM research.

He appears internationally on radio and TV. He is a Founding Diplomate of the American Board of Holistic Medicine; Coordinator for the Council for Healing, a non-profit organization that promotes awareness of spiritual healing; and has served for many years on the advisory boards of the journals, Alternative Therapies in Health and Medicine, Subtle Energies (ISSSEEM), Frontier Sciences, the Advisory Council of the Association for Comprehensive Energy Psychotherapy (ACEP), Emotional Freedom Techniques (EFT) and the Advisory Board of the Research Council for Complementary Medicine (UK), Core reviewer for BioMed Central, Complementary and Alternative Medicine – On line.

Dr. Benor offers introductory telephone tutorials and workshops of 2-8 hours for WHEE.

DB@WholisticHealingResearch.com
www.WholisticHealingResearch.com
www.ijhc.org